HECKMAN'S NURSING PHARMACOLOGY SIMPLIFIED

BY DAVID HECKMAN, PHARMD

**HECKMAN'S
NURSING PHARMACOLOGY SIMPLIFIED**

HECKMAN'S
NURSING PHARMACOLOGY SIMPLIFIED

DISCLAIMERS & COPYRIGHT

Heckman's Nursing Pharmacology Simplified

ISBN-13: 978-1942682110
ISBN-10: 1942682115

Medical information and best practices are constantly changing. The author has attempted to provide accurate, up to date information at the time of publication. Due to constant changes and the potential for human error, the accuracy of the information in this publication cannot be guaranteed. The author, publisher, and all other parties involved in the production of this publication make no warranty (express or implied) regarding the information contained herein.

The author, publisher, and all other parties involved in the production of this book do not assume and hereby disclaim any liability to any party for loss, injury, damage, and/or failure resulting from an error or omission, regardless of cause.

Readers are advised to review the package insert from the manufacturer before administering any drug. It is the responsibility of the reader to verify all information and take appropriate safety precautions when utilizing any information in practice. The author, publisher, and all other parties involved in the production of this book do not assume and hereby disclaim any liability to any party for consequences from the use of this information

This publication is intended for entertainment purposes only and does not constitute medical, legal, or professional advice. The reader is advised to obtain the services of a competent professional for all matters. This publication is not intended to be used, nor should it be used, to diagnose or treat any medical condition.

Copyright © 2018 by David Heckman. All rights reserved. This book is protected by copyright. No portion of this book may be reproduced in any form or by any means including mechanical, electronic, photocopying, scanning, recording, or otherwise without prior express written permission from the author.

Printed in the United States of America.

HECKMAN'S NURSING PHARMACOLOGY SIMPLIFIED

TABLE OF CONTENTS

BACTERIAL INFECTIONS
- Nitroimidazole Antibiotics 9
- Penicillin Antibiotics 10
- Cephalosporin Antibiotics 11
- Nitrofuran Antibiotics 12
- Lincosamide Antibiotics 13
- Macrolide Antibiotics 14
- Tetracycline Antibiotics 15
- Aminoglycoside Antibiotics 16
- Glycopeptide Antibiotics 17
- Fluoroquinolone Antibiotics 18
- Sulfonamide-Folate Antagonist 19
- Oxazolidinone Antibiotics 20

FUNGAL INFECTIONS
- Azole Antifungals 21

VIRAL INFECTIONS
- Herpes Antivirals 22
- Influenza Antiviral 23
- Antiretrovirals 24

CANCER
- Taxanes 25
- Vinca Alkaloids 26
- Folate Antagonist 27
- Topoisomerase I Inhibitors 28
- Anthracyclines 29
- Platinum Complexes 30
- Nitrogen Mustards 31

ANEMIA
- Erythropoiesis-Stimulating Agents 32
- Iron Supplements 33

BONE & JOINT
- Bisphosphonates 34
- Anti-Gout Agents 35

IMMUNE SYSTEM
- Tumor Necrosis Factor Blockers 36
- Calcineurin Inhibitors 37
- Antihistamines 38

PULMONARY
- Inhaled Beta$_2$ Agonists 39
- Inhaled Anticholinergics 40
- Inhaled Corticosteroids 41
- Leukotriene Receptor Antagonists 42
- Methylxanthines 43

NERVOUS SYSTEM
- Anticholinergics 44
- Acetylcholinesterase Inhibitors 45
- Dopamine Precursor 46
- Dopamine Agonists 47
- Antiepileptic Drugs 48
- Gabapentinoids 49
- Barbiturates 50
- Benzodiazepines 51
- Non-Benzodiazepine Sedative-Hypnotics 52
- Muscle Relaxants 53
- Central Nervous System Stimulants 54

HECKMAN'S
NURSING PHARMACOLOGY SIMPLIFIED

- Selective Serotonin Reuptake Inhibitors 55
- Serotonin-Norepinephrine Reuptake Inhibitors 56
- Norepinephrine-Dopamine Reuptake Inhibitors 57
- Tricyclic Antidepressants 58
- Monoamine Oxidase Inhibitors 59
- Triptans 60
- Typical Antipsychotics 61
- Atypical Antipsychotics 62
- Prokinetic-Antiemetic 63
- 5-HT$_3$ Receptor Antagonists 64

GASTROINTESTINAL
- Laxatives 65
- Antidiarrheals 66
- Antacids 67
- Proton Pump Inhibitors 68
- H2 Receptor Antagonists 69
- Gastrointestinal Protectants 70
- Prostaglandin Analogs 71

ENDOCRINE
- Insulin 72
- Biguanides 73
- Oral Hypoglycemic Agents 74
- GLP-1 Agonists 75
- Synthetic Thyroid Hormone 76
- Antithyroid Drugs 77
- Androgens 78
- 5-Alpha Reductase Inhibitors 79
- Combination Hormone Contraceptives 80
- Progestin-Only Contraceptives 81
- Aromatase Inhibitors 82
- Glucocorticoids 83
- Mineralocorticoids 84

CARDIOVASCULAR
- Loop Diuretics 85
- Thiazide Diuretics 86
- Potassium-Sparing Diuretics 87
- ACE Inhibitors and ARBs 88
- Beta-Blockers 89
- Alpha-Blockers 90
- Alpha$_2$ Agonists 91
- Calcium Channel Blockers 92
- Organic Nitrates 93
- PDE-5 Inhibitors 94
- Antiarrhythmics 95
- Digitalis Glycosides 96
- Potassium chloride 97
- Vasopressors 98
- Vitamin K Antagonists 99
- Oral Direct Thrombin Inhibitors 100
- Oral Factor Xa Inhibitors 101
- Heparin 102
- Thienopyridines 103
- Bile Acid Resins 104
- HMG-CoA Reductase Inhibitors 105
- Fibrates 106

PAIN
- Non-Steroidal Anti-Inflammatory Drugs 107
- Coal Tar-Derived Analgesics 108
- Opioid Analgesics 109

DEDICATION

To Grandma Bert Heckman, for showing us how to suck it up and get things done. After attending nursing school at Memorial Hospital in Pawtucket, RI, she joined the Army Nurse Corps with a classmate and was assigned overseas to the 112th Evacuation Hospital during World War II. Upon returning to the United States, she worked as a registered nurse at Greenville Hospital and eventually became the first Director of Nurses at St. Paul Homes in Greenville, PA. Love you, Grandma!

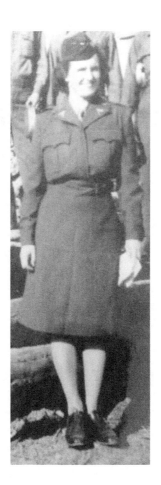

START HERE

HECKMAN'S
NURSING PHARMACOLOGY SIMPLIFIED

NITROIMIDAZOLE ANTIBIOTICS

THE MOST COMMON EXAMPLE
Flagyl® (metronidazole)

Mechanism: Metronidazole enters the microorganism and gains electrons from electron transport proteins in anaerobic pathogens. Upon receiving electrons, metronidazole becomes a highly reactive free radical that destroys vital cellular components like DNA, ultimately leading to cell death.
Common Uses: Anaerobic bacterial and protozoal infections

BACTERICIDAL

BLACK BOX WARNING: POTENTIALLY CARCINOGENIC
Metronidazole was carcinogenic in animal studies. This medication should be used only when necessary.
NOTE: There is no evidence that normal doses significantly increase the risk of cancer in humans.

NO ALCOHOL
WHILE TAKING *and for* THREE DAYS AFTER FINISHING METRONIDAZOLE
Combining alcohol with metronidazole can cause an Antabuse® (disulfiram)-like reaction such as nausea/vomiting, abdominal cramps, flushing, and headaches.

THE MOST COMMON *and* SERIOUS SIDE EFFECTS
The most common side effects can be categorized broadly as "gastrointestinal (GI) side effects," and the most serious side effects as "central nervous system (CNS) side effects."

GI	CNS
COMMON SIDE EFFECTS	**SERIOUS SIDE EFFECTS**
Nausea/Vomiting, Metallic Taste, Dry Mouth, Diarrhea, Abdominal Cramps	Seizures, Aseptic Meningitis, Peripheral & Optic Neuropathy, Encephalopathy

IMPORTANT EDUCATION POINTS *for* ALL ANTIBIOTICS
#1 Antibiotics should only be used for bacterial infections. They are not effective for viral infections.
#2 To prevent development of antibiotic-resistant bacteria, patients should finish the entire prescribed course of antibiotics. Advise patients not to discontinue the antibiotics early, even if they feel better.
#3 In killing pathogenic bacteria, antibiotics also kill good bacteria (flora), including the good bacteria that normally colonize the GI tract. This commonly results in diarrhea, nausea, and vomiting–the most common side effects of antibiotics–and potential overgrowth of *Clostridium difficile* leading to *C. difficile*-associated diarrhea (CDAD), which can be potentially fatal. Notify the physician if the patient develops symptoms of CDAD, such as watery and/or bloody stools.
#4 Intestinal flora produce vitamin K that is absorbed into the bloodstream, so antibiotics can be expected to reduce vitamin K levels. In the presence of less vitamin K, warfarin exerts a stronger anticoagulant effect that can lead to serious bleeding events. For patients on warfarin, monitor INR closely and anticipate an increase.

NOTE: The four points described above apply to **all antibiotics** (pages 9–20).
EXCEPTION: Because *C. difficile* is an anaerobe, metronidazole is actually used to treat *C. difficile* infections.

HECKMAN'S
NURSING PHARMACOLOGY SIMPLIFIED

PENICILLIN ANTIBIOTICS

COMMON EXAMPLES
1st Generation (Natural Penicillins): penicillin V, penicillin G
2nd Generation (Antistaphylococcal Penicillins): nafcillin, methicillin, oxacillin, dicloxacillin
3rd Generation (Aminopenicillins): amoxicillin, ampicillin
4th Generation (Antipseudomonal Penicillins): piperacillin, ticarcillin

Drug Name Stem: –cillin
Mechanism: Penicillins inhibit bacterial cell wall synthesis.
Common Uses: Infections caused by susceptible bacteria (mostly gram-positive)

BACTERICIDAL

ALLERGIC REACTIONS
Penicillins are known for causing allergic reactions such as rash (common) and anaphylaxis (rare).

NO MRSA COVERAGE
None of the penicillins are effective against methicillin-resistant *Staphylococcus aureus* (MRSA).

SEIZURES
Seizures can occur with high doses of penicillins, especially in patients with renal failure.

BETA-LACTAMASE INHIBITORS
Bacteria commonly develop resistance to penicillins by producing beta-lactamases—enzymes that destroy the chemical structure of beta-lactam antibiotics like penicillins, rendering them inactive. This type of resistance can be overcome by administering penicillin-beta lactamase inhibitor combinations. Examples include Augmentin® (amoxicillin/clavulanate), Unasyn® (ampicillin/sulbactam), and Zosyn® (piperacillin/tazobactam).

NOTE: *The spectrum of antibacterial activity is the key differentiator between generations. The chart below provides a basic overview of some major differences in coverage.*

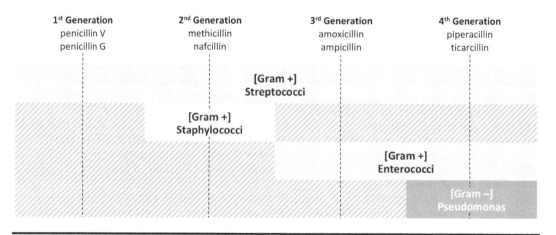

IMPORTANT EDUCATION POINTS *for* ALL ANTIBIOTICS
#1 Only use antibiotics for bacterial infections. **#2** Finish the entire course of antibiotics as prescribed.
#3 Notify physician of watery and/or bloody stools. **#4** For patients on warfarin, monitor INR closely.

HECKMAN'S
NURSING PHARMACOLOGY SIMPLIFIED

CEPHALOSPORIN ANTIBIOTICS

COMMON EXAMPLES
1st Generation Cephalosporins: Keflex® (cephalexin), Ancef® (cefazolin)
2nd Generation Cephalosporins: Ceftin® (cefuroxime), Ceclor® (cefaclor)
3rd Generation Cephalosporins: Omnicef® (cefdinir), Rocephin® (ceftriaxone)
4th Generation Cephalosporins: Maxipime® (cefepime)
5th Generation Cephalosporins: Teflaro® (ceftaroline)

Drug Name Stem: ceph–, cef–
Mechanism: Cephalosporins inhibit bacterial cell wall synthesis.
Common Uses: Infections caused by susceptible bacteria

BACTERICIDAL

UP TO 10% CROSS-REACTIVITY WITH PENICILLINS
Up to 10% of patients with a penicillin allergy may also exhibit an allergy to cephalosporins. History of **severe allergy** to penicillin (e.g. anaphylaxis) generally precludes the use of cephalosporins.

SEIZURES
As with penicillins, seizures can occur with high doses of cephalosporins, especially in patients with renal failure.

NOT EFFECTIVE for ENTEROCOCCI
Unlike the penicillins, none of the cephalosporins possess any clinically useful activity against enterococci.

NOTE: *The spectrum of antibacterial activity is the key differentiator between generations. The chart below provides a basic overview of some major differences in coverage.*

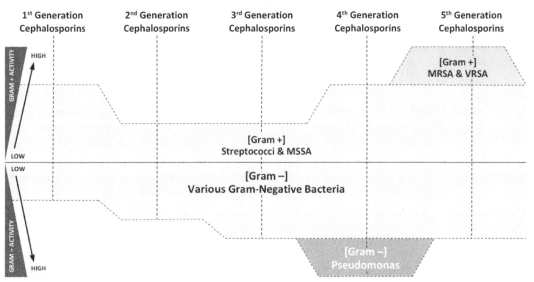

Abbreviations: MRSA, methicillin-resistant *S. aureus*; VRSA, vancomycin-resistant *S. aureus*; MSSA, methicillin-sensitive *S. aureus*.

IMPORTANT EDUCATION POINTS for ALL ANTIBIOTICS
#1 Only use antibiotics for bacterial infections. #2 Finish the entire course of antibiotics as prescribed.
#3 Notify physician of watery and/or bloody stools. #4 For patients on warfarin, monitor INR closely.

HECKMAN'S
NURSING PHARMACOLOGY SIMPLIFIED

NITROFURAN ANTIBIOTICS

COMMON EXAMPLE
MacroBid®, Macrodantin® (nitrofurantoin)

Mechanism: Bacterial enzymes reduce (add electrons to) nitrofurantoin, forming highly reactive intermediates that destroy bacterial macromolecules, such as ribosomes and DNA. This interrupts several vital processes and ultimately leads to bacterial cell death.

Common Uses: Uncomplicated urinary tract infections (UTIs) caused by susceptible strains of *Escherichia coli* or *Staphylococcus saprophyticus*

BACTERICIDAL

⊃ ADMINISTER WITH FOOD ⊂
Administering nitrofurantoin with food increases absorption by 40% and potentially reduces the incidence of nausea.

NITROFURANTOIN COMMONLY CAUSES HARMLESS BROWN DISCOLORATION *of the* URINE

COMMON MINOR SIDE EFFECTS	RARE SERIOUS SIDE EFFECTS
Nausea, Headache, Flatulence	Pulmonary Fibrosis/Pneumonitis, Neuropathy

URINARY TRACT INFECTIONS

Nitrofurantoin must be highly concentrated to exert its antimicrobial effect. Effective concentrations can only be reached in the urine. For this reason, nitrofurantoin is only effective for infections of the lower urinary tract. Furthermore, for the drug to concentrate in the urine, the kidneys must be functioning normally. Significant renal impairment (e.g. creatinine clearance < 60 mL/min) is a contraindication for nitrofurantoin.

MACROBID® *for* TREATMENT	MACRODANTIN® *for* PROPHYLAXIS
Macrobid® is given twice daily (BID) for treatment of UTIs.	Macrodantin® is given once daily (QD) at bedtime for prevention of UTIs.

NOTE: Macrodantin® can be given four times daily (QID) for **treatment** of UTIs; however, this is rarely done in practice since Macrobid® provides the same benefit with BID dosing.

IMPORTANT EDUCATION POINTS *for* ALL ANTIBIOTICS
#1 Only use antibiotics for bacterial infections. **#2** Finish the entire course of antibiotics as prescribed.
#3 Notify physician of watery and/or bloody stools. **#4** For patients on warfarin, monitor INR closely.

HECKMAN'S
NURSING PHARMACOLOGY SIMPLIFIED

LINCOSAMIDE ANTIBIOTICS

THE MOST COMMON EXAMPLE
Cleocin® (clindamycin)

Mechanism: Clindamycin binds to the 50S ribosomal subunit, which is only found in bacterial cells, inhibiting bacterial protein synthesis.

Common Uses: Serious Streptococcal*, Pneumococcal*, Staphylococcal*, or anaerobic bacterial infections
*For gram-positive infections, clindamycin is typically reserved for patients who are allergic to penicillin.

BACTERIOSTATIC

BLACK BOX WARNING
for CLOSTRIDIUM DIFFICILE-ASSOCIATED DIARRHEA

Nearly every antibiotic comes with the risk of C. difficile-associated diarrhea (CDAD), but none has a stronger link to CDAD than clindamycin. For this reason, clindamycin is the only antibiotic that carries a **black box warning** for CDAD. It should be reserved for serious infections that cannot be treated appropriately with other less toxic antibiotics.

NOTE: Instruct patients to notify their healthcare provider if they develop watery and/or bloody stools. This is likely a sign of CDAD and may occur two or more months after finishing a course of antibiotics. The risk of CDAD is greater in elderly patients (age 65+).

PARENTERAL ADMINISTRATION of CLINDAMYCIN

IV
MAXIMUM 30 MG/MIN INFUSION RATE
Rapid intravenous (IV) infusion rates > 30 mg/minute are associated with hypotension and cardiopulmonary arrest. Never administer clindamycin undiluted as an IV bolus.

IM
MAXIMUM 600 MILLIGRAMS PER INJECTION
Intramuscular (IM) injections can cause irritation, pain, induration and sterile abscess. To avoid these side effects, administer the injection deep into the muscle and do not exceed 600 mg per injection.

IMPORTANT EDUCATION POINTS for ALL ANTIBIOTICS
#1 Only use antibiotics for bacterial infections. #2 Finish the entire course of antibiotics as prescribed.
#3 Notify physician of watery and/or bloody stools. #4 For patients on warfarin, monitor INR closely.

**HECKMAN'S
NURSING PHARMACOLOGY SIMPLIFIED**

MACROLIDE ANTIBIOTICS

COMMON EXAMPLES
Zithromax®, Z-pak® (azithromycin)   Biaxin® (clarithromycin)   Ery-Tab® (erythromycin)

Mechanism: Macrolides inhibit protein synthesis in susceptible bacteria by binding to the 50S subunit of bacterial ribosomes.

Common Uses: Mild–moderate infections caused by susceptible gram-positive, gram-negative, and atypical bacteria

BACTERIOSTATIC

THE MOST COMMON SIDE EFFECTS *of* MACROLIDE ANTIBIOTICS
Nausea/vomiting, diarrhea, and abdominal pain

THE MOST SERIOUS SIDE EFFECTS *of* MACROLIDE ANTIBIOTICS

LIVER TOXICITY	CARDIAC ARRHYTHMIAS
Macrolides can cause severe and fatal liver function abnormalities. Monitor for jaundice, dark urine, nausea, appetite loss, abdominal pain, fatigue, and fever.	More likely in patients who are elderly, have a history of cardiac arrhythmias, take other drugs that can cause arrhythmias, or have an uncorrected electrolyte imbalance.

KEY POINTS REGARDING AZITHROMYCIN

THE MOST COMMONLY PRESCRIBED MACROLIDE	**ADMINISTRATION WITH RESPECT TO ANTACIDS**
Azithromycin is the most commonly prescribed macrolide. It is available in a 5-day pack (Z-pak®) in which the patient takes 500 mg by mouth on day 1, followed by 250 mg daily on days 2–5.	Oral azithromycin should not be administered at the same time as antacids that contain aluminum and magnesium hydroxide, as these products can interfere with absorption.

MINIMUM 1-HOUR INTRAVENOUS INFUSION TIME
A 2-mg/mL intravenous (IV) infusion of azithromycin should be administered over no less than 60 minutes. More rapid infusions are associated with IV infusion site reactions.

IMPORTANT EDUCATION POINTS *for* ALL ANTIBIOTICS
#1 Only use antibiotics for bacterial infections. **#2** Finish the entire course of antibiotics as prescribed.
#3 Notify physician of watery and/or bloody stools. **#4** For patients on warfarin, monitor INR closely.

HECKMAN'S
NURSING PHARMACOLOGY SIMPLIFIED

TETRACYCLINE ANTIBIOTICS

COMMON EXAMPLES
Monodox® (doxycycline monohydrate)   Vibramycin® (doxycycline hyclate)   Sumycin® (tetracycline)

Mechanism: Tetracyclines inhibit protein synthesis in susceptible bacteria by binding to the 30S subunit of bacterial ribosomes.

Common Uses: Infections caused by susceptible gram-positive, gram-negative, and atypical microorganisms

BACTERIOSTATIC

ESOPHAGEAL INFLAMMATION & ULCERATION
PATIENTS MAY AVOID BY TAKING WITH A FULL GLASS OF WATER & REMAINING UPRIGHT
Tetracyclines can cause esophageal inflammation and ulceration. This occurs when the medication has prolonged contact with the esophagus. Consequently, we can reduce the incidence of esophageal irritation by having our patients wash down the medication with a full glass of water and remain upright for ≥ 60 minutes.

Al^{3+} Mg^{2+} Zn^{2+} $Fe^{2+/3+}$ Ca^{2+}
INTERACTION WITH POLYVALENT CATIONS
Tetracyclines bind to polyvalent cations, forming an insoluble complex that cannot be absorbed from the gastrointestinal tract, effectively rendering the drug inactive. For this reason, when administered orally, tetracyclines should be separated from products that contain polyvalent cations (e.g. antacids, multivitamins, mineral supplements) by at least two hours. When administering tetracyclines intravenously, do not administer the drug through the same intravenous line as polyvalent cations such as calcium or magnesium.

DISCOLORATION *of* THE TEETH
AN IRREVERSIBLE SIDE EFFECT IN PATIENTS ≤ 8 YEARS OLD
As mentioned above, tetracyclines bind to calcium (Ca^{2+}). This includes the calcium in bone-forming tissue. If a patient is exposed to a tetracycline antibiotic during the period of tooth development (between the second half of pregnancy to age 8), permanent discoloration of the teeth can occur. For this reason, tetracyclines should only be used in pregnant women and patients ≤ 8 years old when other options are inappropriate.

TETRACYCLINES MAY REDUCE *the* EFFECT *of* ORAL CONTRACEPTIVES

THE DIFFERENCE BETWEEN MONOHYDRATE *and* HYCLATE
Doxycycline is available in two salt forms, doxycycline hyclate and doxycycline monohydrate. The biggest difference is the monohydrate form dissolves slower and, consequently, tends to cause less gastrointestinal irritation/stomach upset. Otherwise, these two forms of doxycycline are considered equal.

IMPORTANT EDUCATION POINTS *for* ALL ANTIBIOTICS
#1 Only use antibiotics for bacterial infections. #2 Finish the entire course of antibiotics as prescribed.
#3 Notify physician of watery and/or bloody stools. #4 For patients on warfarin, monitor INR closely.

AMINOGLYCOSIDE ANTIBIOTICS

COMMON EXAMPLES
gentamicin   tobramycin   amikacin
NOTE: The injectable formulations are only available generically.

Mechanism: Aminoglycosides inhibit protein synthesis in susceptible bacteria by binding to the 30S subunit of bacterial ribosomes.

Common Uses: Serious infections caused by susceptible gram-negative bacteria, including Pseudomonas

---

BACTERICIDAL

NARROW THERAPEUTIC INDEX
MONITOR DRUG SERUM CONCENTRATIONS
Serum drug concentrations should be monitored periodically. Prolonged elevations in peak and/or trough concentrations increase the risk of toxic effects.

NEPHROTOXICITY
ALMOST ALWAYS REVERSIBLE
Aminoglycosides are well-known for their propensity to impair kidney function. They also rely on the kidneys for elimination from the body. Kidney function should be monitored periodically.

OTOTOXICITY
IRREVERSIBLE/PERMANENT
Aminoglycosides are also known to damage the eighth cranial nerve, which can cause permanent hearing loss and/or loss of balance. Monitoring with serial audiograms is recommended.

NEUROMUSCULAR BLOCKADE
Aminoglycosides can cause neuromuscular blockade and respiratory paralysis. The risk is higher in patients receiving anesthesia, neuromuscular blockers, and/or large transfusions of citrate-anticoagulated blood.
NOTE: Neuromuscular blockade can be reversed by an injection of calcium salts.

THE IMPORTANCE *of* HYDRATION
The risk of toxicity is greater in patients who are dehydrated. On a related note, potent diuretics (furosemide and ethacrynic acid) should be avoided in patients who are being treated with aminoglycosides.

INTRAMUSCULAR & INTRAVENOUS
EFFECTIVE ROUTES *of* ADMINISTRATION *for* SYSTEMIC ACTIVITY
Aminoglycosides are poorly absorbed from the gastrointestinal tract. They are only effective when administered intramuscularly (IM) or intravenously (IV).

IMPORTANT EDUCATION POINTS *for* ALL ANTIBIOTICS
#1 Only use antibiotics for bacterial infections. **#2** Finish the entire course of antibiotics as prescribed.
#3 Notify physician of watery and/or bloody stools. **#4** For patients on warfarin, monitor INR closely.

HECKMAN'S
NURSING PHARMACOLOGY SIMPLIFIED

GLYCOPEPTIDE ANTIBIOTICS

THE MOST COMMON EXAMPLE
Vancocin® (vancomycin)

Mechanism: Glycopeptides inhibit cell wall synthesis by susceptible gram-positive bacteria.

Common Uses: Used parenterally to treat serious or severe infections caused by susceptible strains of gram-positive bacteria, including methicillin-resistant *Staphylococcus aureus* (MRSA), particularly when other antibiotics are resistant or otherwise inappropriate. Can also be used orally for treatment of pseudomembranous colitis caused by *Clostridium difficile* or staphylococcal enterocolitis.

BACTERICIDAL

NARROW THERAPEUTIC INDEX
MONITOR TROUGH LEVELS
Trough levels should be monitored periodically. Blood draws should occur just before (within 30 minutes) administering the next dose of vancomycin to obtain accurate trough level measurements. Prolonged high troughs increase the risk of toxic effects, and low troughs deliver an inadequate antibiotic effect.

NEPHROTOXICITY
Vancomycin can impair kidney function yet relies on the kidneys for elimination. Monitor renal function. Toxicity is more likely when used with other nephrotoxic drugs (e.g. aminoglycosides).

OTOTOXICITY
Vancomycin can also cause permanent hearing loss. Monitoring with serial audiograms may be helpful. Toxicity is more likely when used with other ototoxic drugs (e.g. aminoglycosides).

ADMINISTER INFUSIONS SLOWLY
OVER A PERIOD *of* AT LEAST 60 MINUTES
Rapid infusion of vancomycin is associated with red man syndrome (also known as "red neck syndrome"), an adverse reaction characterized by extreme flushing of the skin on the upper body. Rapid infusion can also cause anaphylactoid reactions including hypotension, urticaria, and difficulty breathing. To avoid these reactions, vancomycin infusions should be administered slowly over at least 60 minutes.

NOTE: Large doses (> 1 gram) should generally be infused over a longer period (> 60 minutes).

ORAL ADMINISTRATION *of* VANCOMYCIN
Vancomycin has a large molecular structure that is poorly absorbed when given orally. For this reason, when treating systemic infections, vancomycin must be given by intravenous infusion; however, vancomycin can be used orally to treat local intestinal infections such as pseudomembranous colitis caused by *C. difficile*.

IMPORTANT EDUCATION POINTS *for* ALL ANTIBIOTICS
#1 Only use antibiotics for bacterial infections. **#2** Finish the entire course of antibiotics as prescribed.
#3 Notify physician of watery and/or bloody stools. **#4** For patients on warfarin, monitor INR closely.

HECKMAN'S
NURSING PHARMACOLOGY SIMPLIFIED

FLUOROQUINOLONE ANTIBIOTICS

COMMON EXAMPLES
Cipro® (ciprofloxacin)   Levaquin® (levofloxacin)   Avelox® (moxifloxacin)

Drug Name Stem: –floxacin

Mechanism: Fluoroquinolones inhibit DNA gyrase and topoisomerase IV to interfere with DNA replication in susceptible bacteria.

Common Uses: Infections caused by susceptible gram-positive, gram-negative, and atypical microorganisms

---

BACTERICIDAL

IMPACT ON THE TENDONS
Fluoroquinolones can cause irreversible damage to the tendons in the form of tendonitis and/or tendon rupture. Patients aged ≥ 60 years, patients on corticosteroids; and patients with kidney, heart, or lung transplants are at a higher risk of having tendon-related issues.

IMPACT ON THE NERVOUS SYSTEM
Fluoroquinolones can trigger seizures or at least lower the seizure threshold. These medications can cause adverse effects related to the nervous system such as dizziness, anxiety, paranoia, hallucinations, nightmares, and insomnia and may cause irreversible peripheral neuropathy.

IMPACT ON THE HEART
Fluoroquinolones can prolong the QT interval, potentially causing life-threatening cardiac arrhythmias. This is more likely in patients who are elderly, have a history of cardiac arrhythmias, have an uncorrected electrolyte imbalance, or take other drugs that can cause arrhythmias.

TYPICAL DOSING INTERVAL

Cipro® (ciprofloxacin)	Levaquin® (levofloxacin)	Avelox® (moxifloxacin)
Every 12 Hours (BID)	Every 24 Hours (QD)	Every 24 Hours (QD)

INTERACTION WITH POLYVALENT CATIONS
When administered orally, fluoroquinolones should not be given within several hours of other agents that contain polyvalent cations such as aluminum (Al^{3+}), magnesium (Mg^{2+}), zinc (Zn^{2+}), iron (Fe^{2+}/Fe^{3+}), or calcium (Ca^{2+}). When given intravenously, do not administer through the same line as polyvalent cations.

ADMINISTER INFUSIONS OVER 60 MINUTES
Administer slowly. Rapid infusions are associated with hypotension.
NOTE: High-dose levofloxacin (750 mg) should be infused over a period of 90 minutes.

IMPORTANT EDUCATION POINTS *for* ALL ANTIBIOTICS
#1 Only use antibiotics for bacterial infections. **#2** Finish the entire course of antibiotics as prescribed. **#3** Notify physician of watery and/or bloody stools. **#4** For patients on warfarin, monitor INR closely.

HECKMAN'S
NURSING PHARMACOLOGY SIMPLIFIED

SULFONAMIDE-FOLATE ANTAGONIST

THE ONLY EXAMPLE
Bactrim®, Septra® (sulfamethoxazole/trimethoprim)
NOTE: Abbreviations for sulfamethoxazole/trimethoprim include SMZ/TMP, TMP/SMZ, and TMP/SMX.

Mechanism: Sulfamethoxazole (a sulfonamide antibiotic) blocks dihydropteroate synthetase, a key enzyme involved in the bacterial production of folic acid. Trimethoprim (a folate antagonist) selectively inhibits bacterial dihydrofolate reductase, a key enzyme involved in the metabolic activation of folic acid. Without folic acid, bacterial DNA replication and protein synthesis cannot occur, and the bacteria die.

Common Uses: Urinary tract infections, otitis media, shigellosis (a type of traveler's diarrhea), *Pneumocystis jirovecii* pneumonia*, and other infections caused by susceptible bacteria
* Formerly known as *"Pneumocystis carinii* pneumonia."

BACTERICIDAL

ADMINISTER INTRAVENOUS INFUSIONS OVER 60–90 MINUTES
NOTE: Never administer sulfamethoxazole/trimethoprim by intramuscular injection.

STAY WELL-HYDRATED
Sulfamethoxazole is poorly soluble. Crystalluria and ureteral stones can develop, particularly in patients who are dehydrated. Advise patients to drink plenty of fluids while taking sulfamethoxazole/trimethoprim.

SEVERE ADVERSE REACTIONS

BONE MARROW DEPRESSION
Monitor complete blood count periodically.

SKIN REACTIONS
If a rash develops, notify the physician.

HYPERKALEMIA
Monitor serum potassium levels.

POTENTIAL *for* BIRTH DEFECTS WHEN USED DURING PREGNANCY
While trimethoprim does not interfere with the activity of folic acid in normal human cells, it may interfere with folic acid activity in the developing fetus. The use of sulfamethoxazole/trimethoprim during the **first trimester** may increase the risk of congenital malformations such as neural tube defects.

DO NOT ADMINISTER SULFAMETHOXAZOLE TO PATIENTS WITH A SULFA ALLERGY

IMPORTANT EDUCATION POINTS *for* ALL ANTIBIOTICS
#1 Only use antibiotics for bacterial infections. **#2** Finish the entire course of antibiotics as prescribed.
#3 Notify physician of watery and/or bloody stools. **#4** For patients on warfarin, monitor INR closely.

HECKMAN'S
NURSING PHARMACOLOGY SIMPLIFIED

OXAZOLIDINONE ANTIBIOTICS

THE MOST COMMON EXAMPLE
Zyvox® (linezolid)

Mechanism: Oxazolidinones inhibit protein synthesis in susceptible bacteria by binding to the 50S subunit of bacterial ribosomes.

Common Uses: Infections caused by susceptible gram-positive bacteria, including streptococci, staphylococci, and enterococci

---

BACTERIOSTATIC against staphylococci and enterococci.
BACTERICIDAL against streptococci.

ZYVOX® (LINEZOLID) COVERS MRSA & VRE
Linezolid covers two of the most difficult-to-treat drug-resistant gram-positive bacteria, methicillin-resistant *Staphylococcus aureus* (MRSA) and vancomycin-resistant *Enterococcus faecium* (VRE).

MONITOR COMPLETE BLOOD COUNT (CBC) WEEKLY
Linezolid can suppress production of red blood cells, white blood cells, and platelets. This can lead to conditions such as anemia, leukopenia, pancytopenia, and thrombocytopenia. Monitor CBC weekly.

LINEZOLID INHIBITS MONOAMINE OXIDASE
AND CREATES CONCERNS SIMILAR TO MONOAMINE OXIDASE INHIBITORS (MAOIs)

Avoid OTC decongestants and foods/beverages that are rich in tyramine. *	Never administer linezolid within 2 weeks of a monoamine oxidase inhibitor.	Avoid use with serotonin-enhancing drugs like SSRIs, TCAs, and triptans.
↓	↓	↓ ↓
TO AVOID HYPERTENSIVE CRISIS		TO AVOID SEROTONIN SYNDROME

See page 54 for a summary of tyramine-rich foods and beverages.

↑ BLOOD PRESSURE
Zyvox® (linezolid) use may increase blood pressure. Monitor blood pressure periodically.

NERVE DAMAGE ESPECIALLY WHEN USED *for* PERIODS *of* 4+ WEEKS
When used for extended periods (4+ weeks), Zyvox® (linezolid) can cause peripheral and optic neuropathy. Instruct patients to report to their physician if they develop numbness or tingling in the hands and feet, blurred vision, or other vision changes. Optic neuropathy could progress to complete loss of vision.

IMPORTANT EDUCATION POINTS *for* ALL ANTIBIOTICS
#1 Only use antibiotics for bacterial infections. **#2** Finish the entire course of antibiotics as prescribed.
#3 Notify physician of watery and/or bloody stools. **#4** For patients on warfarin, monitor INR closely.

HECKMAN'S
NURSING PHARMACOLOGY SIMPLIFIED

AZOLE ANTIFUNGALS

COMMON EXAMPLES
Diflucan® (fluconazole)   Nizoral® (ketoconazole)

Drug Name Stem: –azole
NOTE: Do not confuse with "–prazole" (the drug name stem for proton pump inhibitors).

Mechanism: Azole antifungals block a cytochrome P450 enzyme involved in the production of ergosterol, a vital component of fungal cell walls, ultimately causing defects in the fungal cell wall, leakage of intracellular contents, and subsequent fungal cell death.

Common Uses: Candidiasis and other infections caused by susceptible species of fungi

DRUG INTERACTIONS
DUE TO INHIBITION of CYTOCHROME P450

As discussed above, the azole antifungals inhibit a cytochrome P450 enzyme. The problem is, cytochrome P450 enzymes are not unique to fungal cells. Humans also rely on cytochrome P450 enzymes, predominantly located in the liver, for metabolism and biosynthesis of various chemicals. Drugs that rely on cytochrome P450 enzymes for metabolism are generally dosed on the assumption that the patient's cytochrome P450 enzymes are functioning at full capacity. For patients taking azole antifungals, this is typically not the case. When the azole antifungal inhibits an enzyme that normally metabolizes another drug, the drug can accumulate and reach toxic levels in the bloodstream. For one example (among many others), the elimination of certain HMG-CoA reductase inhibitors ("statins"), particularly simvastatin and lovastatin, relies on cytochrome P450 enzymes. When these enzymes are inhibited, the statin can accumulate in the bloodstream and dramatically increase the risk of serious adverse effects such as rhabdomyolysis.

HEPATOTOXICITY
A SERIOUS POTENTIAL ADVERSE REACTION

Azole antifungals are associated with rare, but severe and potentially fatal hepatotoxicity. Monitoring of liver function tests is recommended. Also watch for signs of liver dysfunction, such as jaundice.

NAUSEA
THE #1 SIDE EFFECT of AZOLE ANTIFUNGALS
Other common side effects include vomiting, headache, diarrhea, and abdominal pain.

DIFLUCAN® (FLUCONAZOLE)
for TREATMENT of VAGINAL CANDIDIASIS
Fluconazole is commonly prescribed as a one-time dose for the treatment of vaginal candidiasis or "yeast infections." Candida is a type of yeast, and yeast is a type of fungus.

TOPICAL KETOCONAZOLE
GENERALLY, NO SYSTEMIC SIDE EFFECTS
Topical antifungals aren't well-absorbed through the skin, so we don't worry about systemic side effects like hepatotoxicity when administering antifungals topically.

HECKMAN'S
NURSING PHARMACOLOGY SIMPLIFIED

HERPES ANTIVIRALS

COMMON EXAMPLES
Valtrex® (valacyclovir)   Zovirax® (acyclovir)

Drug Name Stem: –vir

Mechanism: Inhibits DNA polymerase/incorporates into viral DNA.

Common Uses: Herpes labialis (cold sores), genital herpes, varicella (chickenpox), herpes zoster (shingles)

ACYCLOVIR VERSUS VALACYCLOVIR

Valtrex® (valacyclovir) is merely acyclovir with a valine amino acid molecule attached to enhance absorption. Once absorbed, an enzyme in the bloodstream removes valine, yielding acyclovir.

COMMON SIDE EFFECTS

Headache, nausea/vomiting, and diarrhea

RENAL FAILURE* & NEUROTOXICITY

The most serious side effects of acyclovir and valacyclovir are renal failure and neurotoxicity, both of which are more likely to occur in elderly patients and patients with pre-existing renal impairment who are taking high doses of acyclovir or valacyclovir.

*Dehydration and/or use in combination with other nephrotoxic medications increases the risk of renal failure.

STRATEGIES *for* REDUCING THE RISK *of* RENAL FAILURE

H_2O
MAINTAIN ADEQUATE HYDRATION
Because dehydration increases the risk of renal failure, patients receiving acyclovir or valacyclovir should be instructed to maintain adequate hydration.

1 HOUR
MINIMUM INFUSION TIME
Rapid infusion of Zovirax® (acyclovir) increases the risk of renal failure, so remember to administer acyclovir infusions at a constant rate over at least 1 hour.

INFLUENZA ANTIVIRALS

THE MOST COMMON EXAMPLE
Tamiflu® (oseltamivir)

Drug Name Stem: –vir

Mechanism: Influenza antivirals inhibit the viral enzyme neuraminidase, interfering with the release of viral particles from the host cell membrane.

Common Uses: Treatment and prevention of influenza A & B

TAMIFLU® *for* TREATMENT/PREVENTION

TREATMENT DOSE
75 mg twice daily (BID) for 5 days*

PREVENTION DOSE
75 mg once daily (QD) for 10 days*

*For adults with normal renal function. Dose adjustments are required for patients with impaired renal function. Dosing for children is based on weight.

START WITHIN 48 HOURS *of* SYMPTOM ONSET

For the best results, Tamiflu® (oseltamivir) should be initiated within 48 hours of the onset of symptoms (when used for treatment) or within 48 hours following close contact with an infected person (when used for prevention).

NAUSEA/VOMITING
Nausea/vomiting is the most common side effect of Tamiflu® (oseltamivir).

ADMINISTER WITH FOOD
To decrease the incidence of nausea/vomiting, administer Tamiflu® (oseltamivir) with food.

SERIOUS ADVERSE REACTIONS (RARE)

ANAPHYLAXIS *and* SERIOUS SKIN REACTIONS
Instruct patients to seek immediate medical attention if they develop a skin rash or allergic symptoms. Anaphylaxis and life-threatening skin reactions (e.g. Stevens-Johnson syndrome) may occur.

BEHAVIOR CHANGES IN PEDIATRIC PATIENTS
Monitor for behavior changes and confusion, particularly in children receiving Tamiflu® (oseltamivir). In rare cases, this has led to fatal self-injury.

HECKMAN'S NURSING PHARMACOLOGY SIMPLIFIED

ANTIRETROVIRALS

HUMAN IMMUNODEFICIENCY VIRUS (HIV)
THE 4 MAJOR STEPS *of* HIV REPLICATION THAT ARE TARGETS *of* DRUG THERAPY
STEP 1: Fusion – HIV binds to CD4 receptors and CCR5 co-receptors on the surface of T cells (white blood cells).
STEP 2: Reverse Transcription – Once inside the cell, HIV reverse transcriptase makes viral DNA from viral RNA.
STEP 3: Viral DNA Integration – Integrase incorporates newly formed viral DNA into the DNA of the host T cell.
STEP 4: Viral Assembly – Infected DNA is used to make viral proteins that are assembled to form new HIV viruses.

Fusion Inhibitors	CCR5 Co-Receptor Antagonists
Fuzion® (enfuvirtide)	Selzentry® (maraviroc)
Mechanism: Fusion inhibitors block **STEP 1** by preventing HIV from binding to CD4 receptors on the surface of T cells.	**Mechanism:** CCR5 co-receptor antagonists block **STEP 1** by preventing HIV from binding to CCR5 co-receptors on T cells.
Nucleoside Reverse Transcriptase Inhibitors (NRTIs)	**Non-nucleoside Reverse Transcriptase Inhibitors (NNRTIs)**
Viread® (tenofovir) Retrovir® (zidovudine)	Sustiva® (efavirenz) Viramune® (nevirapine)
Mechanism: NRTIs block **STEP 2** by mimicking nucleosides, causing reverse transcriptase to incorporate NRTIs into the viral DNA, which ultimately halts viral DNA synthesis.	**Mechanism:** NNRTIs block **STEP 2** by binding to and deactivating reverse transcriptase, which ultimately prevents the process of viral DNA synthesis from occurring.
Integrase Strand Transfer Inhibitors (INSTIs)	**Protease Inhibitors (PIs)**
Isentress® (raltegravir) Tivicay® (dolutegravir)	Norvir® (ritonavir) Prezista® (darunavir)
Mechanism: INSTIs block **STEP 3** by inhibiting the integrase enzyme, preventing viral DNA from being integrated into the T cell DNA.	**Mechanism:** PIs block **STEP 4** by inhibiting protease, the enzyme that cleaves viral proteins, allowing them to be assembled into new HIV viruses.

Drug Name Stem: -vir-

THE FUNDAMENTALS *of* ANTIRETROVIRAL THERAPY

USE A COMBINATION *of* ANTIRETROVIRALS
HIV is notorious for developing drug resistance. To reduce the likelihood of resistance, most patients are on two or more different antiretrovirals.

STRESS THE IMPORTANCE *of* COMPLIANCE
Poor compliance greatly increases the likelihood that HIV will develop resistance mechanisms and the medications will become ineffective.

THE BACKBONE *of* HIV THERAPY
NRTIs are the "backbone" of HIV therapy. Regimens commonly include two NRTIs.

KEY MONITORING PARAMETERS
✓Viral Load   ✓CD4 Count

ANTIRETROVIRALS DO NOT CURE HIV
Antiretrovirals can reduce viral load and prevent HIV from destroying the immune system, but they do not cure HIV. Advise patients with HIV to avoid unprotected sex and sharing needles.

TAXANES

COMMON EXAMPLES
Taxotere® (docetaxel) Taxol® (paclitaxel)

Drug Name Stem: –taxel

Mechanism: Microtubule movement is essential to cell division. Taxanes bind to and stabilize microtubules, preventing their movement and ultimately inhibiting cell division.

Common Uses: Certain cancers (e.g. breast, lung, prostate, gastric, and head/neck)

BONE MARROW SUPPRESSION
THE MAJOR DOSE-LIMITING TOXICITY *of* TAXANES

This can manifest as low white blood cell counts (neutropenia, leukopenia), low red blood cell counts (anemia), and/or low platelet counts (thrombocytopenia). In particular, monitor the neutrophil count. An absolute neutrophil count (ANC) of 1,500 cells/mm^3 is the lower limit of the normal range. Generally, taxanes should not be administered to patients with an ANC below 1,500 cells/mm^3; otherwise, severe neutropenia and infection may occur.

GENERAL RULE: DO NOT ADMINISTER *if* ANC < 1,500

OTHER COMMON SIDE EFFECTS
Alopecia (hair loss), peripheral neuropathy, liver impairment, nausea/vomiting, diarrhea, and weakness/lack of energy

---

PRE-MEDICATE ALL PATIENTS
TO PREVENT HYPERSENSITIVITY REACTIONS WITH TAXANES

Severe and potentially fatal hypersensitivity reactions (e.g. hypotension, difficulty breathing, angioedema) can occur with the administration of taxanes. For this reason, all patients receiving a taxane should receive a corticosteroid (e.g. dexamethasone) prior to administration.

NOTE: Patients receiving Taxol® (paclitaxel) should also receive antihistamines (e.g. diphenhydramine and ranitidine) prior to the infusion.

POLYETHYLENE-LINED TUBING
TO PREVENT EXPOSING PATIENTS TO THE PLASTICIZER (DEHP)

Some infusion administration sets are made of plasticized polyvinyl chloride (PVC). The plasticizer is DEHP. When lipophilic fluid comes into contact with PVC, the plasticizer DEHP is released into the fluid. This is dangerous because DEHP has many potentially toxic effects, including liver toxicity. Both docetaxel and paclitaxel are highly lipophilic. When administering these infusions, be sure to use polyethylene-lined tubing to reduce the patient's exposure to DEHP.

**ADVISE PATIENTS TO AVOID PREGNANCY BY USING EFFECTIVE CONTRACEPTION
AND TO REFRAIN FROM BREASTFEEDING**

**HECKMAN'S
NURSING PHARMACOLOGY SIMPLIFIED**

VINCA ALKALOIDS

COMMON EXAMPLES
Oncovin® (vincristine)   Velban® (vinblastine)

Drug Name Stem: vin–

Mechanism: Microtubules, which are essential to cell division, are formed from tubulin. Vinca alkaloids prevent tubulin from assembling into microtubules, ultimately inhibiting cell division.

Common Uses: Hodgkin's disease, non-Hodgkin's lymphoma, acute leukemia, solid tumors

---

FOR INTRAVENOUS USE ONLY
POTENTIALLY FATAL *if* GIVEN BY OTHER ROUTES
Inadvertent intrathecal administration will likely result in ascending paralysis and death.

THE DOSE-LIMITING TOXICITIES
Cancer chemotherapy drugs are notoriously toxic not only to cancer cells, but to normal cells as well. Consequently, many of these drugs have adverse effects that can be so severe that they may make it necessary to discontinue or otherwise change the treatment plan.

NEUROTOXICITY
DOSE-LIMITING TOXICITY *of* VINCRISTINE
This typically develops progressively, first manifesting as sensory impairment and paresthesia, then neuropathic pain, and finally motor dysfunction. If motor dysfunction occurs, the dose may need to be reduced or discontinued.

LEUKOPENIA
DOSE-LIMITING TOXICITY *of* VINBLASTINE
Vinca alkaloids can cause bone marrow suppression. White blood cell production is most commonly affected. Check a complete blood count before each dose. If leukopenia occurs, monitor closely for signs of infection.

EXTRAVASATION
Vinca alkaloids should only be administered by experienced individuals. The needle or catheter must be properly placed prior to injecting. When vinca alkaloids leak into the surrounding tissue (extravasation), they can cause severe irritation. This is one reason why vinca alkaloids should never be given by subcutaneous or intramuscular injection. If extravasation occurs, the infusion should be stopped, and the remaining dose should be administered into a different vein.

TREATING EXTRAVASATION *of* VINCA ALKALOIDS
Local injection of hyaluronidase in the area of extravasation.
Application of moderate heat to the area of extravasation.

HAIR LOSS
A COMMON SIDE EFFECT *of* VINCA ALKALOIDS
Hair loss (alopecia) is not permanent. Regrowth typically begins even with continued maintenance therapy.

**ADVISE PATIENTS TO AVOID PREGNANCY BY USING EFFECTIVE CONTRACEPTION
AND TO REFRAIN FROM BREASTFEEDING**

FOLATE ANTAGONIST

THE MOST COMMON EXAMPLE
Trexall® (methotrexate)

Mechanism: Methotrexate inhibits dihydrofolate reductase, a key enzyme involved in the metabolic activation of folic acid, ultimately interfering with DNA synthesis in rapidly dividing cells and lymphocytes.

Common Uses: Rheumatoid arthritis (RA), psoriasis, certain cancers (e.g. lymphoma, breast cancer)

ADMINISTERED ONCE WEEKLY
for RA and PSORIASIS
To avoid unintentional overdoses by patients using methotrexate for RA or psoriasis, it is crucial to ensure they understand the dose should be taken just **once weekly**. Accidental daily use of methotrexate can be deadly.

THE TOXIC EFFECTS *of* METHOTREXATE
Rapidly proliferating cells such as cancer cells, fetal cells, gastrointestinal mucosa, and bone marrow are particularly sensitive to the effects of methotrexate. Consequently, we can expect issues like teratogenicity (see below) and side effects like nausea/vomiting, diarrhea, ulcerative stomatitis (mouth sores), and bone marrow suppression. Furthermore, methotrexate is toxic to the liver and has the potential to precipitate in the kidneys, causing acute renal failure. Laboratory monitoring (e.g. complete blood count, serum creatinine, liver function tests) to detect bone marrow, liver, and kidney toxicities is required at baseline and once every 1–2 months.

MONITOR *for* DRY COUGH
Development of a dry, nonproductive cough during treatment with methotrexate can be a sign of a serious pulmonary lesion, which may warrant discontinuation of therapy and further investigation.

PREGNANCY CATEGORY X
Methotrexate can cause fetal malformations and death. It should never be used in pregnant women for RA or psoriasis; however, the benefit may outweigh potential risks when treating cancer.

ADVISE PATIENTS TO AVOID OVER-THE-COUNTER NSAIDs
Non-Steroidal Anti-Inflammatory Drugs (NSAIDs) can decrease renal perfusion, potentially impairing kidney function. Most methotrexate is excreted renally. When used concurrently, NSAIDs may reduce the elimination rate of methotrexate, increasing the risk of toxicity. Patients should consult a physician before using NSAIDs.

THE ANTIDOTE *for* METHOTREXATE
Leucovorin, a folic acid analog.

HECKMAN'S
NURSING PHARMACOLOGY SIMPLIFIED

TOPOISOMERASE I INHIBITORS

COMMON EXAMPLES
Camptosar® (irinotecan)   Hycamtin® (topotecan)

Mechanism: Topoisomerase I is an enzyme that temporarily breaks strands of DNA during DNA replication. Topoisomerase I inhibitors bind to the topoisomerase I-DNA complex and prevent breaks in DNA from being repaired, effectively destroying DNA, particularly in rapidly dividing cells.

Common Uses: Colon cancer (irinotecan); cervical, ovarian, and small cell lung cancer (topotecan)

BONE MARROW SUPPRESSION
Bone marrow suppression is a potential dose-limiting toxicity of Camptosar® (irinotecan) and Hycamtin® (topotecan). If a patient's absolute neutrophil count (ANC) drops below 1,000 cells/mm³, the dose should be held until the ANC rises above 1,000 cells/mm³. Other blood cell counts should also be monitored, and therapy may need to be adjusted based on the results.

NOTE: Aside from blood counts, also monitor for fever, other signs of infection, and bleeding.

MONITOR *for* NEW OR WORSENING COUGH/DIFFICULTY BREATHING
A new or worsening cough or difficulty breathing can be a sign of potentially fatal interstitial lung disease, which may warrant discontinuation of therapy and further investigation.

SEVERE DIARRHEA
A UNIQUE AND POTENTIAL DOSE LIMITING TOXICITY OF CAMPTOSAR® (IRINOTECAN)

EARLY DIARRHEA	LATE DIARRHEA
Diarrhea that occurs within 24 hours of administration ("early diarrhea") is often accompanied by other cholinergic symptoms such as salivation, lacrimation, and sweating and can be treated or prevented by administering 0.25–1mg of atropine intravenously.	Diarrhea that occurs more than 24 hours after administration ("late diarrhea") can be treated with Imodium® (loperamide), fluid, and electrolytes as needed. Late diarrhea can be life-threatening, leading to dehydration, electrolyte imbalances, intestinal ulceration, and sepsis.

NOTE: To help remember this side effect, associate the drug name "irinotecan" with "I ran to the can."

OTHER COMMON SIDE EFFECTS
Nausea/vomiting and alopecia (hair loss)

TREATING EXTRAVASATION *of* TOPOISOMERASE I INHIBITORS
Flush the affected site with sterile water and apply ice.

ADVISE PATIENTS TO AVOID PREGNANCY BY USING EFFECTIVE CONTRACEPTION AND TO REFRAIN FROM BREASTFEEDING

HECKMAN'S
NURSING PHARMACOLOGY SIMPLIFIED

ANTHRACYCLINES

COMMON EXAMPLES
Adriamycin® (doxorubicin)   Cerubidine® (daunorubicin)   Idamycin® (idarubicin)

Drug Name Stem: –rubicin

Mechanism: Anthracyclines bind to DNA and inhibit nucleic acid synthesis and mitosis, and they induce mutagenic and chromosomal aberrations, particularly in rapidly dividing cells such as cancer cells.

Common Uses: Leukemia, lymphoma, solid tumors

CARDIOTOXICITY
THE CUMULATIVE DOSE-LIMITING TOXICITY *of* ANTHRACYCLINES
Anthracyclines are uniquely and notoriously known to damage heart tissue. Over time, this can cause potentially fatal heart failure, cardiac arrhythmias, or other serious heart conditions. Monitor cardiac function by measuring left ventricular ejection fraction prior to treatment and periodically during treatment.

NOTE: Zinecard® (dexrazoxane) can be administered within 30 minutes prior to Adriamycin® (doxorubicin) to prevent cardiac damage in breast cancer patients who are receiving high cumulative doses of doxorubicin.

BONE MARROW SUPPRESSION
ANOTHER POTENTIALLY DOSE-LIMITING TOXICITY *of* ANTHRACYCLINES
Anthracyclines can cause severe bone marrow suppression. The patient's complete blood count should be monitored closely, as a low white blood cell count can lead to deadly infection and a low platelet count can lead to deadly bleeding events.

EXTRAVASATION
Anthracyclines should only be administered by experienced individuals. The needle or catheter must be properly placed prior to injecting. When vinca anthracyclines leak into the surrounding tissue (extravasation), they can cause severe tissue necrosis. This is one reason why **anthracyclines should never be administered by subcutaneous or intramuscular injection**. If extravasation occurs, the infusion should be stopped, and the remaining dose should be administered into a different vein.

TREATING EXTRAVASATION *of* ANTHRACYCLINES
Application of ice packs for 30 minutes four times daily (QID) for three days.
Surgical debridement may be necessary in certain cases.

RED-COLORED URINE
A SIDE EFFECT *of* ANTHRACYCLINE THERAPY
When you examine an infusion of anthracycline, you'll notice it is red. Perhaps not surprisingly, anthracyclines can impart a red color on the urine. Inform patients that this is normal and should be expected.

**ADVISE PATIENTS TO AVOID PREGNANCY BY USING EFFECTIVE CONTRACEPTION
AND TO REFRAIN FROM BREASTFEEDING**

HECKMAN'S
NURSING PHARMACOLOGY SIMPLIFIED

PLATINUM COMPLEXES

COMMON EXAMPLES
Platinol® (cisplatin)   Paraplatin® (carboplatin)   Eloxatin® (oxaliplatin)

Drug Name Stem: –platin
Mechanism: Platinum complexes deploy atoms of platinum that bind and form cross-links with DNA, ultimately inhibiting DNA replication and transcription, particularly in rapidly dividing cells such as cancer cells.
Common Uses: Ovarian cancer (cisplatin and carboplatin), testicular cancer (cisplatin), bladder cancer (cisplatin), colon cancer (oxaliplatin)

THE MOST COMMON SIDE EFFECTS of PLATINUM COMPLEXES

NAUSEA and VOMITING
Nearly everyone who receives cisplatin, and most patients who receive another platinum complex experience nausea/vomiting. The incidence is reduced by pre-medicating with a 5-HT$_3$ antagonist (e.g. ondansetron) ± a corticosteroid (e.g. dexamethasone).

BONE MARROW SUPPRESSION
All platinum complexes can suppress the bone marrow, leading to low white blood cell (WBC), red blood cell (RBC), and platelet counts. Low WBC counts can predispose patients to serious infections, low RBC counts can cause anemia, and low platelet counts can lead to serious bleeding.

NEUROPATHY
Neuropathy is a common side effect of all platinum complexes; however, oxaliplatin is the most likely of the platinum complexes to cause neuropathy. Oxaliplatin-associated neuropathy tends to be exacerbated by exposure to cold environments and objects, and typically manifest in the hands, feet, mouth, and throat.

NEPHROTOXICITY	BONE MARROW SUPPRESSION	NEUROPATHY
The Dose Limiting Toxicity of Platinol® (cisplatin) ↓	The Dose Limiting Toxicity of Paraplatin® (carboplatin) ↓	The Dose Limiting Toxicity of Eloxatin® (oxaliplatin) ↓
Administer 1–2 liters of pretreatment intravenous (IV) hydration prior to cisplatin to reduce nephrotoxic effects.	Monitor complete blood count and signs of low WBC counts (e.g. fever/infection) and low platelet counts (e.g. bleeding).	Advise patient to wear warm clothes, drink through a straw, avoid cold beverages/ice, wear gloves to touch cold objects.

ANAPHYLACTIC REACTIONS
All platinum complexes can trigger potentially fatal anaphylactic reactions (e.g. flushing, hypotension, shortness of breath) within minutes of administration. These reactions are typically treated with epinephrine, corticosteroids, and antihistamines. If a patient has a severe allergic reaction, then the drug should be permanently discontinued, and other platinum complexes should not be used in the future.

PREVENTING CISPLATIN OVERDOSE
If a dose of cisplatin exceeds 100 mg/m^2, contact the physician prior to administering. Doses that exceed this threshold are likely to have been ordered and/or prepared erroneously.

ADVISE PATIENTS TO AVOID PREGNANCY BY USING EFFECTIVE CONTRACEPTION AND TO REFRAIN FROM BREASTFEEDING

HECKMAN'S
NURSING PHARMACOLOGY SIMPLIFIED

NITROGEN MUSTARDS

THE MOST COMMON EXAMPLE
Cytoxan® (cyclophosphamide)

Mechanism: Nitrogen mustards bind and form cross-links with DNA, ultimately inhibiting DNA replication and transcription, particularly in rapidly dividing cells such as cancer cells.

Common Uses: Certain cancers (e.g. lymphomas, leukemias, neuroblastoma, retinoblastoma, breast cancer)

ADMINISTER SLOWLY
Rapid administration of cyclophosphamide is associated with several adverse reactions including facial swelling, scalp burning, headache, and nasal congestion.

BONE MARROW SUPPRESSION
THE MAJOR DOSE-LIMITING TOXICITY *of* NITROGEN MUSTARDS
Bone marrow suppression, typically characterized by a low white blood cell count, is the most common dose-limiting toxicity of cyclophosphamide. Thrombocytopenia and anemia are also possible. According to the package insert, cyclophosphamide should not be administered to patients with neutrophils ≤ 1,500 /mm^3 or platelets ≤ 50,000/mm^3. Also, monitor temperature frequently to detect fever and possible infection.

UROTOXICITY
Acrolein, a byproduct of Cytoxan® (cyclophosphamide) metabolism, is a toxic substance that causes urinary tract inflammation and bleeding. Advise patients to notify the physician if their urine turns pink or red. The toxic effects of acrolein can be reduced or prevented with aggressive hydration, forced diuresis, frequent bladder emptying, and Mesnex® (mesna). Mesnex® (mesna) binds and detoxifies acrolein.

NOTE: Do not administer cyclophosphamide to patients with obstructed urinary outflow.

CARDIOTOXICITY
Cyclophosphamide can cause various heart problems, including potentially fatal heart failure and arrhythmias. Advise patients to notify the physician if they experience symptoms such as edema, cough, weight gain or palpitations.

PULMONARY TOXICITY
Cyclophosphamide can also cause various lung problems, including pneumonitis and pulmonary fibrosis. Advise patients to notify the physician if they experience any new or worsening pulmonary symptoms such as cough or difficulty breathing.

RISK *of* INFERTILITY
Temporary or permanent infertility can occur in both males and females who receive cyclophosphamide.

COMMON SIDE EFFECTS *of* NITROGEN MUSTARDS
Nausea/vomiting and alopecia (hair loss)

**ADVISE PATIENTS TO AVOID PREGNANCY BY USING EFFECTIVE CONTRACEPTION
AND TO REFRAIN FROM BREASTFEEDING**

ERYTHROPOIESIS-STIMULATING AGENTS

COMMON EXAMPLE
Epogen®, Procrit® (epoetin alfa)

Mechanism: Erythropoiesis-stimulating agents (ESAs) mimic endogenous erythropoietin, a hormone normally released by the kidneys to stimulate red blood cell production by the bone marrow.

Common Uses: Anemia from chemotherapy, zidovudine, or chronic kidney disease

---

↑ RED BLOOD CELL PRODUCTION

KEY MONITORING PARAMETERS

IRON STATUS
Functional red blood cells cannot be produced without hemoglobin. Iron is a key component of hemoglobin. Check iron status (i.e. transferrin saturation and serum ferritin) before and during therapy with an ESA. Nearly every patient will need an iron supplement at some point during therapy.

HEMOGLOBIN LEVELS
Excessive production of red blood cells can lead to deadly cardiovascular events, such as a heart attack or stroke. Monitor hemoglobin regularly. Epoetin alfa should not be administered if the hemoglobin level is nearing or above 11 g/dL (or 12 g/dL, depending on the indication).

BLOOD PRESSURE
Epoetin alfa can increase blood pressure. Monitor blood pressure before and regularly during treatment with an epoetin alfa. Never administer epoetin alfa to a patient with uncontrolled hypertension.

RISK *for* PATIENTS WITH CANCER
Epoetin alfa is associated with tumor progression and cancer recurrence in patients with cancer. Avoid in patients when the anticipated outcome of chemotherapy is a cure.

RISK *of* SEIZURES
Epoetin alfa is associated with an increased risk of seizures, particularly during the first 90 days of therapy.

GRANULOCYTE COLONY-STIMULATING FACTORS
Drugs like Neupogen® (filgrastim) and Neulasta® (pegfilgrastim) are used to increase the production of **white blood cells**. Though they are not ESAs, they work in a similar fashion by mimicking an endogenous hormone (granulocyte colony-stimulating factor) to stimulate white blood cell production by the bone marrow. They are commonly used to treat neutropenia caused by chemotherapy, bone marrow transplant or radiation.

REFRIGERATE *and* DO NOT SHAKE
Drugs like epoetin alfa, filgrastim, and pegfilgrastim are glycoproteins composed of a relatively delicate sequence of over 160 amino acids. If exposed to temperature extremes or force by vigorous shaking, the amino acid chains can break, rendering the medication inactive.

HECKMAN'S
NURSING PHARMACOLOGY SIMPLIFIED

IRON SUPPLEMENTS

COMMON EXAMPLES
Ferrous fumarate   Ferrous sulfate   Ferrous gluconate

Mechanism: Iron is an essential mineral that is required to produce hemoglobin, the component of red blood cells responsible for transporting oxygen.

Common Uses: Treatment and prevention of iron deficiency anemia

---

IRON SALT FORMS
Iron supplements are commercially available in a variety of salt forms. Common formulations include ferrous gluconate, ferrous sulfate, and ferrous fumarate. The amount of elemental iron varies based on the formulation.

FERROUS GLUCONATE	FERROUS SULFATE	FERROUS FUMARATE
33% elemental iron	20% elemental iron*	11.6% elemental iron

*__EXAMPLE:__ Ferrous sulfate 325 mg contains 65 mg of elemental iron.

ENHANCE ABSORPTION of IRON WITH VITAMIN C (ASCORBIC ACID)
Orally administered iron is poorly absorbed from the gastrointestinal (GI) tract. Absorption can be enhanced by administering iron supplements with a product that contains vitamin C (e.g. orange juice).

CORROSIVE PROPERTIES
Iron is corrosive to the GI mucosa. To avoid ulceration of the mouth and esophagus, advise patients to swallow iron tablets whole with a glass of water and do not suck or chew the tablets.

COMMON SIDE EFFECTS
Due to its corrosive properties, iron commonly causes nausea/vomiting and dyspepsia. Although food interferes with absorption, taking iron with food can decrease the incidence of GI side effects.

CONSTIPATION and DARK, TARRY STOOLS
Iron supplements are well-known to cause constipation and dark, tarry stools, particularly at high doses.

IRON REQUIREMENT DURING PREGNANCY
During pregnancy, the female body produces extra blood to supply oxygen to the fetus. Consequently, the daily iron requirement is higher during pregnancy. To meet this need, most prenatal vitamins contain 27 mg of elemental iron.

IRON OVERDOSE
A LEADING CAUSE OF FATAL POISONING IN CHILDREN
Keep iron-containing products out of reach of children and in a child-resistant container.

THE ANTIDOTE for IRON
Desferal® (deferoxamine), an iron chelating agent that facilitates the urinary excretion of iron.

HECKMAN'S
NURSING PHARMACOLOGY SIMPLIFIED

BISPHOSPHONATES

COMMON EXAMPLES
Actonel® (risedronate)   Boniva® (ibandronate)   Fosamax® (alendronate)

Drug Name Stem: –dronate

Mechanism: Bisphosphonates increase bone mineral density by incorporating into the mineral matrix of bone tissue and inhibiting osteoclast activity.

Common Uses: Osteoporosis treatment and prevention, Paget's disease

---

THE CHALLENGE OF ABSORPTION
For bisphosphonates to exert their effect on bone tissue, they must be absorbed from the gastrointestinal (GI) tract into the bloodstream. This is actually a big challenge. On average, only about 0.6% of an orally administered bisphosphonate is absorbed, and almost anything can interfere with absorption. Even coffee or orange juice, if taken along with alendronate, have been shown to reduce absorption by about 60%.

↓

ADDRESSING THE CHALLENGE
Administer bisphosphonates first thing in the morning on an empty stomach and do not give the patient any food, beverages, supplements, or other medications for at least 30–60 minutes.

ESOPHAGEAL IRRITATION	PREVENTION STRATEGIES
Bisphosphonates are known to irritate the esophagus. This can lead to severe problems including esophagitis, esophageal ulcers, and esophageal erosion.	To minimize esophageal irritation, administer bisphosphonates with a full glass of plain water (6–8 ounces), and instruct the patient to remain upright for at least 30–60 minutes.

PATIENTS MUST NOT SUCK, CHEW, OR ALLOW TABLETS TO DISSOLVE IN THE MOUTH
Instruct the patient to swallow the tablet whole. Just as bisphosphonates irritate the esophagus, they can irritate other GI mucosa, including the inside of the mouth. Sucking, chewing, or otherwise allowing the tablet to dissolve in the mouth can lead to oropharyngeal ulceration.

TYPICALLY ADMINISTERED ONCE WEEKLY

THE MOST COMMON SIDE EFFECTS
Two things we know about bisphosphonates are they increase bone mineral density and they are irritating to the GI mucosa. Unsurprisingly, the most noteworthy side effects can be categorized as "musculoskeletal" and "gastrointestinal."

MUSCULOSKELETAL SIDE EFFECTS	GI SIDE EFFECTS
Bone, joint, and muscle pain	Dyspepsia and abdominal pain
Osteonecrosis of the jaw	Esophageal ulceration and erosion

ANTI-GOUT AGENTS

ZYLOPRIM® (ALLOPURINOL)
Administer **after a meal** to reduce stomach upset.

ULORIC® (FEBUXOSTAT)
Administer **with or without** food.

XANTHINE OXIDASE INHIBITORS
Gout is caused by high uric acid levels in the blood that form into urate crystals. The body's immune system attacks the urate crystals as a foreign invader. Since the urate crystals tend to deposit in the joints, this results in severe joint pain and inflammation. Zyloprim® (allopurinol) and Uloric® (febuxostat) are xanthine oxidase inhibitors. They block the key enzyme responsible for the production of uric acid, ultimately reducing serum uric acid levels to facilitate the dissolution of urate crystals.

RASH
MONITOR FOR SKIN RASH
With these medications, a skin rash may be the first sign of a life-threating reaction.

THE PARADOX
THESE DRUGS CAN TRIGGER A GOUT FLARE
Although used to prevent gout attacks, initiation of these drugs can trigger an acute gout attack. An NSAID and Colcrys® (colchicine) are routinely added to prevent gout flares when a xanthine oxidase inhibitor is initiated.

URIC ACID < 6 MG/DL
DOSES BASED ON SERUM URIC ACID LEVELS
One widely employed strategy to reduce the chance of triggering an acute gout attack is initiating allopurinol or febuxostat at a low dose. The dose should then be increased gradually to achieve a target serum uric acid level of < 6mg/dL.

COLCRYS® (COLCHICINE)
Colcrys® (colchicine) is not a xanthine oxidase inhibitor. The pain and inflammation that occur with gout is due to the immune system response. Colcrys® (colchicine) interferes with the migration of white blood cells into the joint space, ultimately reducing the extent of the immune response and the associated damage to the surrounding tissue. Colcrys® (colchicine) predominantly used for acute gout attacks ("gout flares").

DIARRHEA
THE #1 SIDE EFFECT OF COLCRYS® (COLCHICINE)
As the colchicine dose increases, the incidence of diarrhea increases. Other common side effects include abdominal pain, nausea and vomiting. These can be broadly categorized as gastrointestinal side effects.

**HECKMAN'S
NURSING PHARMACOLOGY SIMPLIFIED**

TUMOR NECROSIS FACTOR BLOCKERS

COMMON EXAMPLES
Humira® (adalimumab)   Enbrel® (etanercept)   Remicade® (infliximab)

Mechanism: Tumor necrosis factor (TNF) blockers bind to and effectively deactivate TNF-alpha, ultimately reducing the release of pro-inflammatory chemical messengers and suppressing immune system activity.

Common Uses: Crohn's disease, ulcerative colitis, rheumatoid arthritis, psoriatic arthritis, plaque psoriasis, ankylosing spondylitis

CONSEQUENCES *of* IMMUNOSUPPRESSION
ASSOCIATED WITH TNF BLOCKERS

↑ RISK *of* INFECTION
Infection is the most common side effect associated with TNF blockers. These infections can be fatal. TNF blockers should not be initiated in patients with an active infection, and patients should receive a tuberculin skin test prior to initiating a TNF blocker.

↑ RISK *of* CANCER
Development of malignancy, such as lymphoma or other types of cancer, is another serious risk associated with the use of TNF blockers. These cancers can be fatal. TNF blockers should be used cautiously in patients with a history of cancer.

NO LIVE VACCINES
for PATIENTS RECEIVING TNF BLOCKERS

In patients who are immunosuppressed, such as those receiving TNF blockers, live vaccines (e.g. MMR vaccine, varicella vaccine) can cause severe and potentially deadly reactions due to uncontrolled replication of the virus. Inactivated vaccines are still safe to administer to patients who are immunosuppressed.

THE TWO-HOUR RULE
for REMICADE® (INFLIXIMAB)

Remicade® (infliximab) commonly causes infusion reactions which can occur during or up to **two hours** after administration. Mild–moderate infusion reactions (e.g. headache, chills, mild fever) can be resolved by lowering the infusion rate. Severe infusion reactions (e.g. major drop in blood pressure, trouble breathing, anaphylaxis) require discontinuation of the infusion. To reduce the incidence of infusion reactions, Remicade® (infliximab) should be administered over a period of at least **two hours**. Additionally, pre-medication with antihistamines, acetaminophen, and/or corticosteroids can reduce the incidence of infusion reactions.

**ADMINISTER REMICADE® (INFLIXIMAB)
OVER A PERIOD *of* AT LEAST 2 HOURS**

**MONITOR *for* INFUSION REACTIONS
for 2 HOURS AFTER ADMINISTRATION**

HUMIRA® (ADALIMUMAB) & ENBREL® (ETANERCEPT) ARE ADMINISTERED BY SUBCUTANEOUS INJECTION

CALCINEURIN INHIBITORS

COMMON EXAMPLES
Gengraf®, Neoral®, Sandimmune® (cyclosporine)   Prograf® (tacrolimus)

Mechanism: Calcineurin inhibitors interfere with the activation and proliferation of T-lymphocytes, ultimately suppressing the immune system.

Common Uses: Prevention of organ rejection in patients with liver, kidney or heart transplants

---

RENAL TOXICITY
Calcineurin inhibitors are associated with renal impairment, hypertension, and hyperkalemia. Monitor renal function (e.g. serum creatinine), blood pressure, and potassium levels periodically.

INFECTIONS AND CANCER
Due to its immunosuppressive effects, the use of calcineurin inhibitors increases susceptibility to all types of infections (bacterial, viral, fungal, and protozoal), and increases the risk of cancer, particularly lymphoma and skin cancers. Monitor complete blood count and advise patients to wear sunscreen.

NO LIVE VACCINES
In patients who are taking immunosuppressants such as calcineurin inhibitors, live vaccines (e.g. MMR, varicella vaccine) can cause severe and potentially deadly reactions due to uncontrolled replication of the virus. Inactivated vaccines are still safe to administer; however, they may have a reduced effect.

ANAPHYLAXIS
TRIGGERED BY CASTOR OIL DERIVATIVES
The **injectable** versions of cyclosporine and tacrolimus contain castor oil derivatives that may trigger anaphylactic reactions in some patients. Monitor continuously for signs and symptoms of an anaphylaxis during the initial 30 minutes of the infusion and then at frequent intervals during the remainder of the infusion. Be prepared to administer epinephrine and oxygen if necessary.

NOTE: Oral dosage forms do not contain castor oil derivatives; therefore, patients who have experienced an anaphylactic reaction with the injectable formulations are not expected to be allergic to oral formulations.

NARROW THERAPEUTIC INDEX
Trough concentrations should be monitored frequently. If levels are too low, transplant organ rejection can occur. If levels are too high, toxicities (e.g. nephrotoxicity) are more likely. For accurate trough level measurement, blood draws should occur just prior to the next dose (within 30 minutes).

NOTE: Because low drug levels are associated with transplant organ rejection, it is extremely important that patients take these medications on a consistent schedule exactly as prescribed.

INSTRUCT PATIENTS TO
AVOID GRAPEFRUIT & GRAPEFRUIT JUICE
Grapefruit (and grapefruit juice) contains furanocoumarins which irreversibly inhibit CYP3A4, a key enzyme involved in the metabolism of cyclosporine and tacrolimus.

HECKMAN'S
NURSING PHARMACOLOGY SIMPLIFIED

ANTIHISTAMINES

COMMON EXAMPLES
1st Generation: Benadryl® (diphenhydramine)   Dramamine® (dimenhydrinate)   Unisom® (doxylamine)
2nd Generation: Allegra® (fexofenadine)   Claritin® (loratadine)   Zyrtec® (cetirizine)

Mechanism: Antihistamines antagonize H_1 receptors, opposing the effects of histamine.

Common Uses: Allergies, insomnia (first-generation antihistamines), motion sickness (dimenhydrinate)

FIRST-GENERATION ANTIHISTAMINES

THE MOST COMMON SIDE EFFECT: DROWSINESS
First-generation antihistamines readily cross the blood-brain barrier (BBB), antagonizing histamine receptors in the central nervous system and causing drowsiness. The link to sedation is so strong that diphenhydramine and doxylamine are marketed as over-the-counter sleep aids under the trade names ZzzQuil® and Unisom®, respectively.

HIGHLY ANTICHOLINERGIC
Aside from their reputation for causing sedation, the first-generation antihistamines are also known for having anticholinergic side effects, such as dry mouth, urinary retention, constipation, and confusion. For this reason, the use of first-generation antihistamines should be avoided in elderly populations when possible.

THERAPEUTICALLY VERSATILE
While anticholinergic effects may be undesirable, particularly for elderly patients, they may be capitalized upon therapeutically in certain situations. For instance, first-generation antihistamines can be used for prevention of motion sickness and treatment of nausea/vomiting and cough.

PARADOXICAL EXCITATION
Antihistamines typically cause sedation; however, rarely patients may experience paradoxical excitation (e.g. insomnia, restlessness, tremor, hallucinations). This type of reaction is more common in children.

SECOND GENERATION ANTIHISTAMINES

THE NON-DROWSY ANTIHISTAMINES
Second-generation antihistamines do not cross the BBB to a significant degree and, consequently, do not cause sedation. Nonetheless, some patients may still experience drowsiness, particularly with high doses. Second-generation antihistamines are marketed as "non-drowsy" and are generally more popular than their first-generation counterparts.

MILDLY ANTICHOLINERGIC
Second-generation antihistamines also have fewer and less severe anticholinergic effects and are the preferred alternative to first-generation antihistamines for elderly patients.

HECKMAN'S
NURSING PHARMACOLOGY SIMPLIFIED

INHALED BETA$_2$ AGONISTS

COMMON EXAMPLES
Short-Acting: Ventolin®, ProAir®, Proventil® (albuterol)   Xopenex® (levalbuterol)
Long-Acting: Foradil® (formoterol)   Serevent® (salmeterol)

Mechanism: Beta$_2$ receptor agonists activate beta$_2$-adrenergic receptors, which are located predominantly in the lungs, resulting in bronchodilation.

Common Uses: Asthma, chronic obstructive pulmonary disease (COPD)

INSTRUCTIONS *for the* PATIENT
1) Shake well   2) Actuate and inhale   3) Hold breath for 10 seconds   4) Wait one minute between puffs

SHORT-ACTING
Short-acting beta$_2$ agonists (e.g. albuterol, levalbuterol) are the gold standard/drug of choice for treatment of severe asthma exacerbations ("asthma attacks").

LONG-ACTING
Long-acting beta$_2$ agonists (e.g. formoterol, salmeterol) are not effective in treating asthma attacks. Instead, they should be used daily for prevention.

ROUTE *of* ADMINISTRATION: ADVANTAGES *and* DISADVANTAGES
Administration by inhalation delivers the drug directly to the site of action (the lungs), which maximizes the therapeutic effect while minimizing side effects. However, for an inhaler to be effective, the patient must be able to press the actuator and inhale deeply at the same time. For patients with poor coordination, attaching a spacer to the mouthpiece can solve this problem.

CARDIOVASCULAR SIDE EFFECTS
Palpitations, chest pain, and tachycardia

Beta$_2$ receptors are located predominantly in the lungs; however, receptor selectivity is never 100%. Some minor beta$_1$ receptor activation occurs at baseline. A greater loss of selectivity occurs as the dose increases, so much so that, according to the package inserts, overdoses may be associated with cardiac arrest and death.

DRUG INTERACTION: BETA AGONISTS + BETA-BLOCKERS
Many patients with asthma or COPD have other medical problems that may require the use of a beta-blocker. Non-selective beta-blockers, like carvedilol and labetalol, antagonize beta$_1$ receptors in the heart *and* beta$_2$ receptors in the lungs. Consequently, these beta-blockers can block the receptors that we are trying to activate with inhaled beta$_2$ agonists. This interaction can be avoided by placing patients with asthma or COPD on a beta$_1$-selective (or "cardioselective") beta-blocker like atenolol or metoprolol.

RECOMMEND WEEKLY CLEANING
When an HFA inhaler appears to be dysfunctional or prematurely empty, the typical culprit is a clog in the opening where the medication exits the mouthpiece. This can be prevented with routine cleaning. Instruct patients to clean their inhaler at least once weekly according to the instructions in the package insert.

DO NOT RECOMMEND THE FLOAT TEST
Multiple studies have demonstrated **no reliable correlation** between how high the metal canister floats in water and the amount of medication inside. Furthermore, water may damage the metal canister. The "float test" should not be recommended as a method to determine the amount of medication in an inhaler.

HECKMAN'S
NURSING PHARMACOLOGY SIMPLIFIED

INHALED ANTICHOLINERGICS

COMMON EXAMPLES
Atrovent® (ipratropium)   Spiriva® (tiotropium)

Mechanism: Inhaled anticholinergics block acetylcholine receptors in the airways, resulting in bronchodilation.

Common Uses: Chronic obstructive pulmonary disease (COPD)

MINIMIZING ANTICHOLINERGIC EFFECTS
Certain anticholinergic effects such as blurred vision, constipation, urinary retention, and confusion can be particularly troublesome for elderly patients. Administration by inhalation allows the drug to be applied directly to the site of action, maximizing the therapeutic effect while minimizing side effects.

DRY MOUTH
THE #1 SIDE EFFECT *of* INHALED ANTICHOLINERGICS
The one anticholinergic effect that is not minimized by an inhaled route of administration is dry mouth. Since inhaled anticholinergics encounter the oral cavity on the way to the lungs, the drying effect on the mouth can be pronounced. To reduce the incidence of dry mouth, instruct the patient to rinse their mouth out with water after each use.

SHORT-ACTING
Atrovent® (ipratropium)

LONG-ACTING
Spiriva® (tiotropium)

FDA-APPROVED *for* MAINTENANCE TREATMENT *of* COPD
The most commonly prescribed inhaled anticholinergics are Atrovent® (ipratropium) and Spiriva® (tiotropium). Atrovent® must be administered four times daily, whereas Spiriva® is only administered once daily.

IPRATROPIUM *for* ASTHMA EXACERBATIONS
The short-acting inhaled anticholinergic ipratropium is frequently used off-label in combination with albuterol for treatment of moderate–severe asthma exacerbations. The combination product is marketed under the brand name DuoNeb® (ipratropium/albuterol).

WARNING *for* SPIRIVA® HANDIHALER®
Do not swallow the capsules that come with the Spiriva® Handihaler® device. The Handihaler® device is designed to puncture the capsule, allowing the powder inside the capsule can be inhaled.

NOTE: Spiriva® capsules are not well-absorbed from the gastrointestinal tract. According to the package insert, only 2–3% of orally administered doses are absorbed into the bloodstream. Consequently, if a capsule is mistakenly administered by mouth, the patient is unlikely to experience any therapeutic or adverse effects.

HECKMAN'S NURSING PHARMACOLOGY SIMPLIFIED

INHALED CORTICOSTEROIDS

COMMON EXAMPLES
Asmanex® (mometasone) Flovent® (fluticasone) Pulmicort® (budesonide)

Mechanism: Inhaled corticosteroids bind to glucocorticoid receptors in the airway, reducing the production of inflammatory mediators and suppressing immune system activity.

Common Uses: Asthma maintenance treatment

HIGHLY EFFECTIVE WITH MINIMAL SIDE EFFECTS
Corticosteroids are the most effective drugs for the treatment of asthma. They are typically reserved for moderate–severe cases. When administered orally, long-term use is associated with a plethora of potentially debilitating side effects such as peptic ulcers, hypertension, hyperglycemia, weight gain, and osteoporosis; however, as with other inhaled formulations, administration by inhalation allows the drug to be applied directly to the site of action, which maximizes the therapeutic effect while minimizing side effects.

STRESS THE IMPORTANCE *of* DAILY USE
Inhaled corticosteroids should be used daily for maintenance treatment. They are effective for preventing symptoms, but they are not effective for treating acute bronchospasm ("asthma attacks"). Missed doses increase the risk of asthma attacks and cause a general worsening of symptoms.

COMMON SIDE EFFECTS
✓Upper respiratory infections ✓Oral thrush ✓Sinusitis

These side effects are logical given that inhaled corticosteroids are immunosuppressants delivered directly into the respiratory tract.

RINSE MOUTH
Inhaled corticosteroids are potent anti-inflammatory drugs. Inevitably, they encounter the oral cavity en route to the lungs, suppressing immune system activity within the oral cavity and opening the door to issues like oral thrush (a fungal infection of the mouth). To reduce the incidence of oral thrush, instruct patients to rinse their mouths out with water after each use.

INHALED CORTICOSTEROID + LONG-ACTING BETA$_2$ AGONISTS
The pathophysiology of asthma includes bronchial smooth muscle constriction, airway inflammation and bronchial hyperresponsiveness. While corticosteroids have potent anti-inflammatory effects, they do not treat the underlying bronchoconstriction. For this reason, inhaled corticosteroids are commonly combined with a long-acting beta$_2$ agonist. Some examples of this are Advair® (fluticasone/salmeterol), Dulera®(mometasone/formoterol), and Symbicort® (budesonide/formoterol).

THE ROLE *of* SHORT-ACTING BETA$_2$ AGONISTS
Corticosteroids are not effective for the treatment of asthma attacks. As always, short-acting beta$_2$ agonists (e.g. albuterol, levalbuterol) are the gold standard/drug of choice for treating severe asthma exacerbations ("asthma attacks").

**HECKMAN'S
NURSING PHARMACOLOGY SIMPLIFIED**

LEUKOTRIENE RECEPTOR ANTAGONISTS

COMMON EXAMPLES
Singulair® (montelukast)   Accolate® (zafirlukast)

Drug Name Stem: -lukast

Mechanism: Montelukast and zafirlukast block leukotriene receptors in the airway, ultimately preventing effects such as airway edema, bronchial smooth muscle contraction (bronchoconstriction), and inflammation.

Common Uses: Asthma maintenance treatment

NOT FOR TREATMENT OF ACUTE ASTHMA ATTACKS
Leukotriene receptor antagonists are not effective for treating acute asthma attacks. They are only effective for treating chronic asthma symptoms and preventing asthma exacerbations. If prescribed for asthma, instruct the patient to take the medication every day, regardless of symptoms.

NOTE: Acute asthma attacks should be treated with an inhaled short-acting beta agonist (i.e. albuterol).

MINOR SIDE EFFECTS
In clinical trials, side effects of leukotriene receptor antagonists were similar to placebo.

MINOR BENEFITS
Leukotriene receptor antagonists are typically prescribed for mild–moderate asthma.

RESPIRATORY INFECTIONS
Respiratory infections are a potential side effect of leukotriene receptor antagonists. This makes sense given that leukotrienes promote inflammation, an immune response, and leukotriene receptor antagonists block the actions of leukotrienes in the airway. Reducing inflammation helps open the airways, but at the expense of some immune function in the respiratory tract.

SINGULAIR® (MONTELUKAST) VERSUS ACCOLATE® (ZAFIRLUKAST)

	Singular® (montelukast)	Accolate® (zafirlukast)
Dosing schedule	Once daily	Twice daily
Administration instructions	Take with or without food	Take on an empty stomach
Potential for drug interactions	Low	Moderate
Potential to impair liver function	No	Yes
Additional FDA-approved uses	Prevention of exercise-induced bronchoconstriction and treatment of allergic rhinitis	None

THE POPULARITY OF SINGULAIR® (MONTELUKAST)
As outlined above, Singulair® (montelukast) has advantages over Accolate® (zafirlukast). As expected, Singulair® (montelukast) is more commonly prescribed.

HECKMAN'S
NURSING PHARMACOLOGY SIMPLIFIED

METHYLXANTHINES

COMMON EXAMPLES
Theo-24® (theophylline)   Norphyl® (aminophylline)

Mechanism: Methylxanthines inhibit phosphodiesterase III & IV and antagonize adenosine receptors, promoting bronchial smooth muscle relaxation and reducing responsiveness to airway stimuli.

Common Uses: Acute bronchospasm, asthma, chronic obstructive pulmonary disease

THEOPHYLLINE VERSUS AMINOPHYLLINE
Aminophylline is essentially two theophylline molecules bound together by ethylenediamine, which is inert. Because ethylenediamine has no pharmacologic activity yet adds mass to the compound, a higher dose of aminophylline is required to achieve the same effect as theophylline.

1.25 mg *of* AMINOPHYLLINE = 1 mg *of* THEOPHYLLINE

NARROW THERAPEUTIC INDEX
The concentration of theophylline in blood must be monitored, and the dose must be adjusted accordingly. Inside the body, aminophylline is broken down to two molecules of theophylline. Consequently, serum theophylline levels must also be monitored in patients taking aminophylline.

THERAPEUTIC RANGE
Therapeutic peak serum concentration: 5–20 mcg/mL
Generally, maintaining theophylline levels from 10–15 mcg/mL provides desired therapeutic effects while reducing the risk of toxicity.

TOXICITY
Theophylline toxicity is characterized by persistent vomiting, intractable seizures, and cardiac arrhythmias. Theophylline toxicity, typically occurring with serum concentration > 20 mcg/mL (peak), is potentially deadly!

RELATIONSHIP TO CAFFEINE	COMMON SIDE EFFECTS
Both theophylline and caffeine are methylxanthines. Consequently, the common side effects seen with theophylline are similar to those seen with caffeine, such as one might experience by drinking one or more strong cups of coffee.	✓ Nausea/vomiting ✓ Diarrhea ✓ Headache ✓ Insomnia ✓ Tachycardia ✓ Tremor

ANTICHOLINERGICS

Anticholinergics oppose acetylcholine, the primary neurotransmitter of the parasympathetic nervous system. The most well-known anticholinergic drug is **atropine**, which can be used to treat bradycardia, reduce salivation during anesthesia and surgery, dilate the pupils, and treat organophosphate poisoning.

ACRONYM	EFFECTS *of* ACETYLCHOLINE	ANTICHOLINERGIC EFFECTS
D	Diarrhea	Constipation
U	Urination	Urinary Retention
M	Miosis (Pinpoint Pupils)	Mydriasis (Dilated Pupils)
B	Bradycardia	Tachycardia
B	Bronchospasm & Bronchorrhea	Bronchial Dilation & Dryness
E	Emesis	Antiemetic
L	Lacrimation	Dry Eye
S	Salivation & Sweating	Dry Mouth & Heat Intolerance

THERAPEUTIC UTILITY *of* ANTICHOLINERGIC EFFECTS

Certain anticholinergic effects may be therapeutically beneficial. For example, patients who experience frequent urges to urinate can benefit from anticholinergic drugs that relax the smooth muscle in the bladder wall. Likewise, patients with irritable bowel syndrome (IBS), a disorder characterized in part by gastrointestinal (GI) cramping, can benefit from anticholinergic drugs that reduce GI motility.

COMMON ANTICHOLINERGICS *and* INDICATIONS

Anticholinergics	GI Tract Spasms and IBS	Bladder Spasms and Overactive Bladder	Parkinsonism and Extrapyramidal Symptoms
Levsin® (hyoscyamine)	✓	✓	✓
Bentyl® (dicyclomine)	✓		
Ditropan® (oxybutynin)		✓	
Detrol® (tolterodine)		✓	
Vesicare® (solifenacin)		✓	
Cogentin® (benztropine)			✓
Artane® (trihexyphenidyl)			✓

CLASSIC ANTICHOLINERGIC SIDE EFFECTS

✓Dry Mouth ✓Dry Eye ✓Urinary Retention ✓Constipation ✓Blurred Vision
✓Tachycardia ✓Heat Intolerance ✓Confusion*

*Apart from interfering with the parasympathetic nervous system, anticholinergics also interfere with cognitive function in the central nervous system. This can cause additional side effects like short-term memory loss (particularly bad for patients with dementia), confusion, disorientation, delirium, and hallucinations.

THE ANTIDOTE *for* ANTICHOLINERGICS
Physostigmine, an acetylcholinesterase inhibitor.

HECKMAN'S
NURSING PHARMACOLOGY SIMPLIFIED

ACETYLCHOLINESTERASE INHIBITORS

COMMON EXAMPLES
Aricept® (donepezil)   Exelon® (rivastigmine)

Mechanism: Acetylcholinesterase inhibitors block the enzyme responsible for breaking down acetylcholine, which effectively increases the concentration and effect of endogenously produced acetylcholine.

Common Uses: Dementia of the Alzheimer's type

ALZHEIMER'S DISEASE and ACETYLCHOLINE
Alzheimer's disease is characterized in part by a deficiency of acetylcholine, a central nervous system neurotransmitter.

MOST COMMON SIDE EFFECTS
Nausea/vomiting and diarrhea

NOTE: These side effects can be broadly classified as "gastrointestinal (GI) side effects."
Replenish fluid and electrolytes to prevent dehydration in patients with vomiting and diarrhea.

ACETYLCHOLINE and DUMBBELS
Acetylcholinesterase inhibitors increase the concentration and effect of acetylcholine in the body. This can be beneficial for patients with dementia related to Alzheimer's Disease, a disease partly characterized by a deficiency in the neurotransmitter acetylcholine. However, acetylcholine is involved in a variety of other processes outside of the brain. Remember the DUMBBELS, the mnemonic for the effects of acetylcholine?

D = Diarrhea   U = Urination   M = Miosis   B = Bradycardia   B = Bronchospasm & Bronchorrhea
E = Emesis   L = Lacrimation   S = Salivation & Sweating

This explains why nausea/vomiting (i.e. "emesis") and diarrhea are some of the most common side effects of Aricept® (donepezil) and Exelon® (rivastigmine). It also helps explain some of the less common side effects such as bradycardia, urinary incontinence, and increased sweating.

DRUG INTERACTION
ACETYLCHOLINESTERASE INHIBITORS + NSAIDs
As described in the DUMBBELS mnemonic, acetylcholine stimulates secretion of various bodily fluids (lacrimation, salivation, sweating). Acetylcholine also stimulates gastric acid secretion. This can irritate the lining of the stomach and predispose patients to non-steroidal anti-inflammatory drug-induced gastric ulcers. For patients taking this combination of medications, monitor for signs and symptoms of GI bleeding.

ACETYLCHOLINESTERASE INHIBITORS AS ANTIDOTES
Physostigmine, the primary antidote for anticholinergics (see page 44), is an acetylcholinesterase inhibitor.

THE ANTIDOTE for ACETYLCHOLINESTERASE INHIBITORS
Atropine, an anticholinergic agent.

HECKMAN'S
NURSING PHARMACOLOGY SIMPLIFIED

DOPAMINE PRECURSOR

THE MOST COMMON EXAMPLE
Sinemet® (carbidopa/levodopa)

Mechanism: Levodopa crosses the blood-brain barrier (BBB) to enter the central nervous system (CNS) where it is converted enzymatically to dopamine.

Common Uses: Parkinson's disease

THE ROLE *of* DOPAMINE IN PARKINSON'S DISEASE
Parkinson's disease is a neurodegenerative disease that involves the death of dopamine-producing neurons in the CNS. There is no cure, but symptoms (e.g. resting tremor, muscle stiffness/rigidity, slow voluntary movements) can be relieved by agents that activate dopamine receptors in the CNS.

CHALLENGES *of* SUPPLEMENTING DOPAMINE IN THE CNS

CHALLENGE #1	CHALLENGE #2
Orally administered dopamine will not cross the blood-brain barrier. ⇩	Levodopa is rapidly converted to dopamine by an enzyme in bloodstream before entering the CNS. ⇩
SOLUTION: Administer levodopa instead, because it will readily cross the BBB.	**SOLUTION:** Inhibit the enzyme that converts levodopa to dopamine in the bloodstream.*

*THE ENZYME INHIBITOR
Carbidopa inhibits the enzyme, DOPA decarboxylase, which converts levodopa to dopamine. Carbidopa does not cross the BBB, so it only blocks the conversion to dopamine outside of the CNS.

THE MOST COMMON SIDE EFFECT: NAUSEA
When levodopa is converted to dopamine outside of the CNS, it can cause nausea. Co-administering carbidopa reduces but does not completely eliminate the incidence of nausea. For patients that experience nausea while taking carbidopa/levodopa, administer the medication with a low-protein snack (e.g. crackers).

DYSKINESIA	PSYCHOSIS *and* HALLUCINATIONS
Levodopa commonly causes dyskinesia (involuntary movements), particularly with long-term treatment. The reasons for this are complex and not fully understood.	Levodopa can also cause psychosis and hallucinations. This aligns with the science indicating that excessive dopamine activity is associated with psychosis (see page 62).

DO NOT ADMINISTER LEVODOPA WITH HIGH-PROTEIN FOODS/BEVERAGES
L-tyrosine ⇨ Levodopa ⇨ Dopamine

The body produces levodopa by making a minor chemical modification to the amino acid L-tyrosine. Both compounds are similar and rely on the same saturable active transport mechanism for absorption from the gastrointestinal tract. When levodopa is given with amino acids like L-tyrosine, they compete, and absorption of levodopa is reduced. Consequently, levodopa should not be given with high-protein foods or beverages.

HECKMAN'S
NURSING PHARMACOLOGY SIMPLIFIED

DOPAMINE AGONISTS

COMMON EXAMPLES
Mirapex® (pramipexole)   Requip® (ropinirole)

Mechanism: Dopamine agonists activate dopamine receptors in the central nervous system.

Common Uses: Parkinson's disease, moderate–severe restless leg syndrome

---

THE MOST COMMON SIDE EFFECT: NAUSEA
Like levodopa (the precursor to dopamine), nausea is the most common side effect of dopamine agonists. Dopamine agonists can be taken with or without food; however, administration with food may reduce the incidence of nausea. Unlike levodopa, absorption of dopamine agonists, such as pramipexole and ropinirole, is unaffected when administered with high-protein foods and beverages.

SIDE EFFECTS SIMILAR TO LEVODOPA

DYSKINESIA*	PSYCHOSIS *and* HALLUCINATIONS*
Dopamine agonists commonly cause dyskinesia (involuntary movements).	Exacerbation of psychosis is possible, and hallucinations are common.

*These and other side effects are much more likely to occur in patients receiving three daily doses for treatment of Parkinson's disease than patients who only receive a once-daily dose 2–3 hours before bedtime for restless leg syndrome.

INCREASE DOSE SLOWLY	DISCONTINUE GRADUALLY
To ensure the patient will tolerate a dopamine agonist well, it is best to start at a low dose and increase the dose slowly until the desired effect is achieved.	Abrupt discontinuation is associated with withdrawal symptoms (e.g. fever, confusion, and muscle stiffness). Advise patients to consult their physician before stopping any medication.

SOMNOLENCE *and* SUDDEN SLEEP EPISODES
Although rare, dopamine agonists have been associated with sudden onset of sleep without warning ("sleep attacks"), possibly even while driving. Warn patients of this possible side effect and instruct them to notify their healthcare provider if they experience excessive daytime drowsiness or a sudden sleep episode.

ADVISE PATIENTS TO AVOID ALCOHOL
Alcohol consumption increases the risk of drowsiness, somnolence, and other side effects associated with dopamine agonists. Advise patients to avoid consuming alcoholic beverages while taking these medications.

ANTIEPILEPTIC DRUGS

Dilantin® (phenytoin)	Depakene® (valproic acid)	Tegretol® (carbamazepine)
MAXIMUM INFUSION RATE ⇩ Do not administer rapidly! The **maximum IV infusion rate is 50 mg/minute**. Rapid infusion increases the risk of severe hypotension and potentially deadly cardiac arrhythmias.	**#1 SIDE EFFECT** ⇩ Nausea/Vomiting Valproic acid irritates the stomach and commonly causes nausea/vomiting. **Administer with food** to decrease the incidence of nausea/vomiting.	**RARE ADVERSE EFFECT** ⇩ Although rare, carbamazepine can cause **aplastic anemia and agranulocytosis**. Monitor for chronic infection, easy bruising, nosebleeds, bleeding gums, and/or severe fatigue.

NARROW THERAPEUTIC INDEX DRUGS
Each of the above is a narrow therapeutic index drug, which means there is a small difference between the amount of medication that will produce a therapeutic effect and the amount that will cause toxic and potentially deadly effects. Consequently, patients taking these medications require periodic blood work to ensure the concentration of medication in the blood is maintained within the therapeutic range.

SERIOUS SKIN REACTIONS	LIVER DAMAGE
Although rare, phenytoin, valproic acid, and carbamazepine are associated with potentially fatal skin reactions (e.g. Stevens-Johnson syndrome and toxic epidermal necrolysis. Report rashes to the physician.	Phenytoin, valproic acid, and carbamazepine are some of the top causes of drug-induced liver injury. Look out for signs/symptoms of liver dysfunction (e.g. elevated liver enzymes, jaundice).

BIRTH DEFECTS
The use of phenytoin, valproic acid, or carbamazepine during pregnancy can cause birth defects; however, a seizure during pregnancy could lead to miscarriage. The benefits of using these agents during pregnancy may outweigh the risks. The mother should be informed of the risks. Of note, valproic acid is the most likely antiepileptic drug to cause birth defects (4× more likely than other agents).

SUICIDAL THOUGHTS *and* BEHAVIOR
Patients who take any antiepileptic drug are almost twice as likely to experience suicidal thoughts or behavior. (Risk of suicidal thoughts or behavior: approximately 1 in 500)

PATIENTS SHOULD NOT DISCONTINUE ABRUPTLY
Compliance is very important with antiepileptic drugs. Abrupt discontinuation can lead to status epilepticus with potentially fatal hypoxia. Advise patients to take these medications exactly as prescribed.

HECKMAN'S
NURSING PHARMACOLOGY SIMPLIFIED

GABAPENTINOIDS

COMMON EXAMPLES
Neurontin® (gabapentin)   Lyrica® (pregabalin)

Drug Name Stem: -gaba-

Mechanism: Gabapentin blocks voltage-gated calcium channels in the central nervous system, slowing the release of excitatory neurotransmitters.

Common Uses: Neuropathic pain, postherpetic neuralgia, seizures, fibromyalgia (pregabalin)

CONTROLLED SUBSTANCE STATUS
Lyrica® (pregabalin) is federally classified as a Schedule V (CV) controlled substance. Gabapentin is not considered to be a controlled substance at the federal level; however, some states (e.g. Kentucky, Tennessee) now recognize gabapentin as a CV controlled substance.

SOMNOLENCE and DIZZINESS
Somnolence and dizziness are the most common side effects of gabapentin and pregabalin. Advise patients not to drive or operate heavy machinery until effects are known.

START LOW and INCREASE SLOWLY
To reduce the incidence of side effects, gabapentinoids should be initiated at a low dose and slowly increased to obtain the desired effect.

TOLERANCE TO SIDE EFFECTS
Inform patients that bothersome side effects like somnolence and dizziness typically resolve on their own within the first 1–2 weeks of use.

ADVISE PATIENTS TO AVOID ALCOHOL and OTHER DEPRESSANTS
As the drug name stem suggests (-gaba-), gabapentinoids share some features with gamma-aminobutyric acid (GABA), including a depressant effect on the central nervous system (CNS). To avoid excessive sedation and potentially life-threatening respiratory depression, patients should avoid other CNS depressants (e.g. alcohol) while taking gabapentin or pregabalin.

SUICIDAL THOUGHTS and BEHAVIOR
Patients taking gabapentin are about twice as likely to experience suicidal thoughts or behavior.*

PATIENTS SHOULD NOT DISCONTINUE ABRUPTLY
Compliance is very important. Abrupt discontinuation may lead to withdrawal seizures.*

*The same concerns as with the antiepileptic drugs discussed on the previous page.

GABAPENTIN INTERACTION WITH ANTACIDS
Wait at least two hours after taking an antacid with aluminum or magnesium (e.g. Maalox®, Mylanta®, Gaviscon®) before administering the next dose of gabapentin.

HECKMAN'S
NURSING PHARMACOLOGY SIMPLIFIED

BARBITURATES

THE MOST COMMON EXAMPLE
Luminal® (phenobarbital)

Drug Name Stem: –barbital

Mechanism: Depresses nervous system activity, likely by potentiating the effects of gamma-aminobutyric acid (GABA).

Common Uses: Seizure disorders, sedation

THE #1 SIDE EFFECT: SEDATION/DROWSINESS
Sedation is the most common side effect. Advise patients to avoid dangerous activities like driving until they know how the medication affects them. Also, instruct patients to avoid alcohol while taking barbiturates.

C-IV CONTROLLED SUBSTANCE
Phenobarbital is a potentially addictive and commonly abused drug.

THERAPEUTIC *and* TOXIC EFFECTS
Drugs with less than a two-fold difference between the therapeutic dose and the lethal dose may be deemed to have a "narrow therapeutic index" according to the FDA's definition. Lethal and therapeutic doses of phenobarbital fall just outside of this two-fold threshold, but it is still potentially dangerous.

DO NOT TAKE MORE THAN PRESCRIBED	DO NOT DISCONTINUE ABRUPTLY
High doses of barbiturates can cause **potentially deadly** central nervous system and respiratory depression. Warn patients not to increase the dose without consulting their physician.	Barbiturate withdrawal is **potentially deadly**. The dose should be reduced gradually. Warn patients not to discontinue a barbiturate without consulting their physician.

ADMINISTER INJECTIONS CAREFULLY
Phenobarbital is highly alkaline (pH > 9) and should **never** be administered into an artery or subcutaneous tissue. Intra-arterial administration can cause gangrene, requiring amputation, and subcutaneous administration can lead to tissue necrosis. Give injections intramuscularly (IM) or intravenously (IV).

INTRAMUSCULAR INJECTIONS	INTRAVENOUS INJECTIONS
To avoid tissue irritation, intramuscular injections should be administered deeply into a large muscle (e.g. gluteal muscle) and no more than 5 mL should be injected in any one site.	To minimize the risk of irritation and possible venous thrombosis, intravenous injections should be administered into a large vein at a slow rate of no more than 60 mg/minute.

MONITOR VITAL SIGNS AFTER ADMINISTERING AN INJECTION OF PHENOBARBITAL

BIRTH DEFECTS
Like phenytoin, valproic acid, and carbamazepine, use of phenobarbital during pregnancy may lead to birth defects; however, a seizure during pregnancy could cause a miscarriage. The benefits of using phenobarbital during pregnancy may outweigh the risks. The mother should be informed of the risks.

BENZODIAZEPINES

COMMON EXAMPLES
Xanax® (alprazolam) Klonopin® (clonazepam) Valium® (diazepam)
Ativan® (lorazepam) Restoril® (temazepam) Halcion® (triazolam)

Drug Name Stems: –azolam, –azepam

Mechanism: Benzodiazepines activate benzodiazepine receptors, enhancing the effect of gamma-aminobutyric acid (GABA), the chief inhibitory neurotransmitter in the central nervous system (CNS).

Common Uses: Anxiety, panic disorders, insomnia, seizures, muscle spasms

WARNING
Benzodiazepines are CNS depressants. Use with other CNS depressants such as opioids, sedatives or alcohol could lead to severe sedation, respiratory depression, coma, and death.

C-IV
CONTROLLED SUBSTANCES
Benzodiazepines have potential for abuse and addiction. Warn patients not to increase the dose without consulting their physician.

2X
RISK of SUICIDALITY
As with any antiepileptic drug, patients are about twice as likely to experience suicidal thoughts or behavior.

THE #1 SIDE EFFECT: DROWSINESS
Drowsiness and other CNS side effects (e.g. dizziness, fatigue) are related to the pharmacological activity of benzodiazepines and typically resolve with continued use as tolerance develops.

PATIENTS SHOULD AVOID IF PREGNANT or BREASTFEEDING
Use during pregnancy may lead to birth defects and neonatal withdrawal symptoms.

PATIENTS SHOULD NOT DISCONTINUE ABRUPTLY
Dependence can develop quickly. Abrupt discontinuation may precipitate withdrawal symptoms, including seizures. Benzodiazepines should be discontinued gradually. Advise patients not to stop taking a benzodiazepine without consulting their physician.

THE ANTIDOTE for BENZODIAZEPINES
Romazicon® (flumazenil), a benzodiazepine receptor antagonist.

HECKMAN'S
NURSING PHARMACOLOGY SIMPLIFIED

NON-BENZODIAZEPINE SEDATIVE-HYPNOTICS

COMMON EXAMPLES
Ambien® (zolpidem)   Sonata® (zaleplon)   Lunesta® (eszopiclone)

Mechanism: Non-benzodiazepine sedative-hypnotics interact with the gamma-aminobutyric acid (GABA)-benzodiazepine receptor complex and enhance the effect of GABA, the chief inhibitory neurotransmitter of the central nervous system (CNS).

Common Uses: Insomnia

NO ALCOHOLIC BEVERAGES
Medications in this drug class are CNS depressants that may impair cognitive and motor function. Patients should not consume alcohol while taking these medications.

C-IV

CONTROLLED SUBSTANCES
Mild potential for abuse, addiction, and dependence.

SLEEP-WALKING *and* OTHER COMPLEX BEHAVIORS
Non-benzodiazepine sedative-hypnotics have been associated with sleep-walking, sleep-driving, making phone calls, and preparing and eating food while not fully awake and with no memory afterward.

SPECIAL ADMINISTRATION INSTRUCTIONS

TAKE WITHOUT FOOD	TAKE IMMEDIATELY BEFORE BED
Do not administer with or immediately after meals. Food has the effect of slowing and reducing absorption of these medications, potentially rendering them ineffective.	Remaining awake after taking these medications leads to an increased probability of experiencing unpleasant side effects like hallucinations and impaired coordination.

DEVOTE A FULL NIGHT TO SLEEP
The sedative-hypnotic effect typically wears off after approximately eight hours or less. Consequently, these medications should only be used when the patient can devote a full night (approximately 7–8 hours) to sleep. Patients should also be warned of the potential for "next-day impairment" (i.e. daytime drowsiness that may preclude them from safely operating a vehicle the day after using the medication).

MOST COMMON SIDE EFFECTS
✓Headache   ✓Drowsiness   ✓Dizziness

WORSENING *of* DEPRESSION
Patients with depression who use these medications should be monitored for worsening of depression and suicidal thoughts or actions.

MUSCLE RELAXANTS

COMMON EXAMPLES
Flexeril® (cyclobenzaprine)   Liorisal (baclofen)   Soma® (carisoprodol)

Mechanism: Muscle relaxants depress central nervous system (CNS) activity.

Common Uses: Relief of muscle spasms/discomfort caused by acute musculoskeletal conditions (cyclobenzaprine, carisoprodol) and relief of muscle spasticity caused by multiple sclerosis (baclofen)

DROWSINESS
THE #1 SIDE EFFECT *of* MUSCLE RELAXANTS
Patients should avoid driving or operating machinery until the effects are known.
Patients must not drink alcohol while taking these medications.

BACLOFEN
STRUCTURALLY RELATED TO GAMMA-AMINOBUTYRIC ACID
The chemical structure of baclofen is similar to that of gamma-aminobutyric acid, the chief inhibitory neurotransmitter of the CNS. This association helps explain why the use of baclofen is associated with side effects like drowsiness, dizziness, weakness, and fatigue.

CYCLOBENZAPRINE
STRUCTURALLY RELATED TO TRICYCLIC ANTIDEPRESSANTS
The chemical structure of cyclobenzaprine is similar to that of the tricyclic antidepressants (TCAs). The big themes with TCAs (see page 58) include drowsiness, cardiovascular side effects (e.g. cardiac arrhythmias), anticholinergic side effects (e.g. dry mouth, constipation, blurred vision, confusion), potential for serotonin syndrome (particularly when combined with other medications that enhance the activity of serotonin), and lowering of the seizure threshold. The same concerns apply to cyclobenzaprine.

CARISOPRODOL
PHARMACOLOGICALLY SIMILAR TO BARBITURATES
Carisoprodol produces effects similar to those of barbiturates, including activation of the reward pathway in the brain, which can lead to addiction and abuse. Consequently, carisoprodol is federally classified as a Schedule IV controlled substance.

POTENTIAL *for* ABUSE
Muscle relaxants, even those that are not controlled substances, can be used by drug abusers to enhance the effect of other CNS depressants. This is particularly dangerous, as it can lead to fatal respiratory depression.

NOTE: Monitor for drug-seeking behavior.

HECKMAN'S
NURSING PHARMACOLOGY SIMPLIFIED

CENTRAL NERVOUS SYSTEM STIMULANTS

COMMON EXAMPLES
Adderall® (amphetamine/dextroamphetamine)   Vyvanse® (lisdexamfetamine)
Ritalin® (methylphenidate)   Concerta® (methylphenidate ER)   Focalin® (dexmethylphenidate)

Mechanism: Central nervous system (CNS) stimulants block the neuronal reuptake and increase the neuronal release of norepinephrine and dopamine.

Common Uses: Attention deficit hyperactivity disorder (ADHD), Narcolepsy

C-II
CONTROLLED SUBSTANCES
Due to their high potential for abuse and addiction, the CNS stimulants reviewed on this page are federally recognized as Schedule II controlled substances.

CARDIOVASCULAR SIDE EFFECTS
Cardiovascular side effects are obvious consequences of enhanced norepinephrine activity.

↑ BLOOD PRESSURE
On average, stimulants raise blood pressure by 2–4 mmHg. Individual patients may experience large increases in blood pressure. Monitor blood pressure periodically.

↑ HEART RATE
On average, stimulants increase heart rate by 3–6 bpm. Individual patients may experience large increases in heart rate. Monitor heart rate periodically.

RISK of CARDIOVASCULAR EVENTS
✓ Heart Attack   ✓ Stroke   ✓ Sudden Death

NOTE: CNS stimulants should generally be avoided in patients with serious heart problems.

CNS SIDE EFFECTS
Stimulants are to depressants as night is to day. Just as depressants such as benzodiazepines, are used to treat anxiety and insomnia, stimulants may cause anxiety and insomnia.

✓ Anxiety   ✓ Insomnia   ✓ Emotional Lability

↓ SEIZURE THRESHOLD
As one might expect from stimulant drugs, CNS stimulants can lower the seizure threshold, making it more likely for seizures to occur. If a patient experiences a seizure, the CNS stimulant should be discontinued.

ADMINISTER IN THE MORNING
Evening or nighttime administration is likely to cause insomnia.

**HECKMAN'S
NURSING PHARMACOLOGY SIMPLIFIED**

SELECTIVE SEROTONIN REUPTAKE INHIBITORS

COMMON EXAMPLES
Prozac® (fluoxetine)   Paxil® (paroxetine)   Zoloft® (sertraline)
Celexa® (citalopram)   Lexapro® (escitalopram)   Desyrel® (trazodone)

Mechanism: Selective serotonin reuptake inhibitors (SSRIs) interfere with neuronal reuptake of serotonin, effectively enhancing the effect of serotonin in the central nervous system (CNS).

Common Uses: Depression, anxiety disorders, bulimia, panic disorder, obsessive compulsive disorder, post-traumatic stress disorder

SEVERAL WEEKS TO PEAK EFFECT
It is important to understand there are no quick fixes for depression.
All antidepressants have a slow onset of action and may require several weeks to reach peak effect.

THE BLOOD, BRAIN, and BOWELS
Serotonin is found predominantly in the gastrointestinal tract ("bowels"), the CNS ("brain"), and platelets ("blood"). Not surprisingly, this is where we see many of the effects of SSRIs, many of which are unwanted.

GASTROINTESTINAL SIDE EFFECTS	NEUROPSYCHIATRIC SIDE EFFECTS
✓Diarrhea ✓Constipation ✓Dry mouth ✓Nausea ✓Dyspepsia ✓Abdominal pain	✓Insomnia ✓Somnolence ✓Dizziness ✓Tremor ✓Decreased libido ✓Anxiety

INCREASED RISK of UPPER GASTROINTESTINAL BLEEDING
Fortunately, the effect of SSRIs on platelets is minor. The primary concern is a small increase in the risk of upper gastrointestinal bleeding. The risk of bleeding increases with the use of non-steroidal antiinflammatory drugs, aspirin, warfarin, and/or other drugs that affect coagulation.

NOTE: Some side effects may seem illogical at first glance. Diarrhea **and** constipation? Insomnia **and** somnolence? In the case of SSRIs, it is best to just focus on the big picture.

MAY IMPAIR COGNITIVE and MOTOR FUNCTION
All psychiatric medications have the potential to impair cognitive and motor function. Advise patients to avoid driving and operating machinery until they know how SSRIs affect them. Also, advise patients to avoid alcohol.

PATIENTS SHOULD NOT DISCONTINUE ABRUPTLY
Adverse effects have been associated with abrupt discontinuation.
To reduce the likelihood of adverse effects, the dose should be reduced gradually when possible.

BLACK BOX WARNING for ANTIDEPRESSANTS
Antidepressant use is associated with an increased risk of suicidality for patients age ≤ 24 years.
Monitor all patients on antidepressants for worsening of depression and suicidal thoughts/behaviors.

NOTE: Use of antidepressants actually decreases the risk of suicidality in patients age ≥65 years.

SEROTONIN-NOREPINEPHRINE REUPTAKE INHIBITORS

COMMON EXAMPLES
Cymbalta® (duloxetine)   Effexor® (venlafaxine)   Pristiq® (desvenlafaxine)
Savella® (milnacipran)   Fetzima® (levomilnacipran)

Mechanism: Serotonin-norepinephrine reuptake inhibitors (SNRIs) interfere with neuronal reuptake of serotonin and norepinephrine, effectively enhancing the effects of serotonin and norepinephrine in the central nervous system (CNS).

Common Uses: Depression, anxiety disorders, diabetic nerve pain, fibromyalgia, chronic pain

---

MAJOR SIMILARITIES TO SSRIs
Selective serotonin reuptake inhibitors (SSRIs) and SNRIs both enhance the effect of serotonin in the CNS by blocking neuronal serotonin reuptake. Logically, this leads to other similarities (see below).

Onset of action	Slow onset of action. May require several weeks to reach peak effect.
Side effects	Predominant side effects are gastrointestinal and neuropsychiatric with a slight increase in the risk of upper gastrointestinal bleeding.
Impairment	May impair cognitive and motor function. Advise patients to avoid driving and operating machinery until they know how the medication affects them. Also, advise patients to avoid alcohol.
Discontinuation	Abrupt discontinuation is associated with adverse effects. The dose should be reduced gradually when possible.
Black box warning	Antidepressants are associated with an increased risk of suicidality in patients ≤ 24 years old. Monitor all patients on antidepressants for worsening of depression and suicidal thoughts/behaviors.

MAJOR DIFFERENCES *from* SSRIs
While SSRIs selectively block the reuptake of serotonin, SNRIs block the reuptake of serotonin **and** norepinephrine. Consequently, SNRIs can have cardiovascular side effects (see below).

HYPERTENSION* | **TACHYCARDIA**

*Monitor blood pressure prior to starting an SNRI and then periodically as treatment continues.

SEROTONIN SYNDROME
Serotonin syndrome is a potentially life-threatening condition characterized by:
mental status changes (e.g. agitation, hallucinations, coma),
autonomic instability (e.g. tachycardia, blood pressure changes, sweating, hyperthermia),
neuromuscular symptoms (e.g. tremor, rigidity, hyperreflexia, incoordination),
gastrointestinal symptoms (nausea/vomiting, diarrhea),
and/or **seizures**.

Serotonin syndrome can occur with the use of a single agent (e.g. an SSRI); however, the risk increases with the use of multiple serotonin-enhancing agents such as SSRIs, SNRIs, tricyclic antidepressants, triptans, and/or St. John's Wort.

NOREPINEPHRINE-DOPAMINE REUPTAKE INHIBITORS

THE MOST COMMON EXAMPLE
Wellbutrin® (bupropion)

Mechanism: Norepinephrine-dopamine reuptake inhibitors (NDRIs) inhibit the neuronal reuptake of norepinephrine and dopamine, effectively enhancing their effects in the central nervous system (CNS).

Common Uses: Depression, smoking cessation

THE HIGHLIGHTS of BUPROPION

THE APPEARANCE of AN INTACT TABLET IN THE STOOL
Some extended-release bupropion tablets have an insoluble outer shell that may show up in the patient's stool. No need to panic. Further investigation will expose this freeloading floater as a mere hollow shell.

RISK of SEIZURES
MAXIMUM DOSE 450 MG PER DAY
Bupropion can cause seizures. The higher the dose, the greater the risk of seizures. Bupropion should never be administered to patients with a history of seizures or certain patients who are predisposed to seizures.

HIGH BLOOD PRESSURE
DUE TO NOREPINEPHRINE ACTIVITY
Like serotonin-norepinephrine reuptake inhibitors, NDRIs work by increasing the effects of norepinephrine. This can lead to elevated blood pressure (BP). Monitor BP prior to starting bupropion and then periodically thereafter.

ZYBAN® (BUPROPION) for SMOKING CESSATION
The NDRI drug class (i.e. bupropion) is unique from other antidepressants in a couple of ways. First, the mechanism of action does not involve serotonin. Second, it is the only antidepressant that is also effective as an aid for smoking cessation.

THE RECURRING THEMES of ANTIDEPRESSANTS

STARTING AN ANTIDEPRESSANT
All antidepressants, including bupropion, have a slow onset of action and may require several weeks to reach peak effect.

STOPPING AN ANTIDEPRESSANT
Abruptly discontinuing antidepressants, including bupropion, can lead to adverse reactions. Reduce the dose gradually when possible.

BLACK BOX WARNING for ANTIDEPRESSANTS
Antidepressant use is associated with an increased risk of suicidality for patients age 24 and under. Monitor all patients receiving an antidepressant, including bupropion, for worsening of depression and suicidal thoughts and/or behaviors.

IMPAIRMENT POTENTIAL
All antidepressants, including bupropion, may impair cognitive and motor function. Patients should avoid driving until the effects are known.

INTERACTION WITH ALCOHOL
Combining alcohol with an antidepressant, including bupropion, can lead to adverse events. Advise patients to avoid alcoholic beverages.

TRICYCLIC ANTIDEPRESSANTS

COMMON EXAMPLES
Elavil® (amitriptyline)   Pamelor® (nortriptyline)
Tofranil® (imipramine)   Silenor® (doxepin)

Mechanism: Tricyclic antidepressants (TCAs) interfere with neuronal reuptake of serotonin and norepinephrine, effectively enhancing the effects of serotonin and norepinephrine in the central nervous system (CNS).

Common Uses: Depression, nerve pain

MAJOR DIFFERENCES *from* SEROTONIN-NOREPINEPHRINE REUPTAKE INHIBITORS (SNRIs)
Looking at the mechanism, one might assume that TCAs are just like SNRIs. While there are similarities, there are also some key differences. For instance, TCAs tend to have more pronounced cardiovascular effects and a variety of anticholinergic effects. For these reasons, TCAs are typically not prescribed unless a patient has failed to respond to the newer antidepressants (e.g. selective serotonin reuptake inhibitors or SNRIs).

A MNEMONIC *for* TRICYCLIC ANTIDEPRESSANTS
Why are TCAs a relatively unpopular class of antidepressants?
Two Reasons: **C**ardiovascular & **A**nticholinergic Side Effects

CARDIOVASCULAR EFFECTS	ANTICHOLINERGIC EFFECTS
Hypertension, Postural Hypotension, Tachycardia, Arrhythmia, Heart Attack, Stroke	Dry Mouth, Blurred Vision, Constipation, Tachycardia, Urinary Retention, Confusion

TRICYCLIC ANTIDEPRESSANTS
LOWER THE SEIZURE THRESHOLD

DROWSINESS	BEDTIME
THE #1 MOST COMMON SIDE EFFECT	**ADMINISTRATION IS TYPICAL**
Drowsiness is the most common side effect; however, patients typically develop tolerance with continued use.	To reduce the incidence of daytime drowsiness, most tricyclic antidepressants should be administered at bedtime.

NOTE: Elderly patients are particularly prone to excessive sedation and confusion with TCAs.

SEROTONIN SYNDROME
Risk of serotonin syndrome increases when multiple serotonin-enhancing agents are used at the same time.

THE RECURRING THEMES *of* ANTIDEPRESSANTS
#1 Expect a slow onset of action (2+ weeks).   **#2** Avoid abrupt discontinuation.
#3 Monitor patients for worsening of depression and suicidal thoughts and/or behaviors.
#4 Avoid driving until the effects are known.   **#5** Avoid alcoholic beverages.

HECKMAN'S
NURSING PHARMACOLOGY SIMPLIFIED

MONOAMINE OXIDASE INHIBITORS

COMMON EXAMPLES
Nardil® (phenelzine)   Parnate® (tranylcypromine)   Marplan® (isocarboxazid)

Mechanism: Monoamine oxidase inhibitors (MAOIs) inhibit the enzyme monoamine oxidase, effectively increasing the concentration of norepinephrine and serotonin in the nervous system.

Common Uses: Depression

ADVISE PATIENTS TO AVOID LARGE AMOUNTS *of* TYRAMINE *and* CAFFEINE
Caffeine is a central nervous system (CNS) stimulant. Tyramine triggers the release of catecholamines (dopamine, norepinephrine, and epinephrine), which are also CNS stimulants. Meanwhile, MAOIs inhibit the breakdown of norepinephrine, a CNS stimulant. Combining MAOIs with large amounts of caffeine and/or tyramine can overload the nervous system with stimulants, causing potentially fatal **hypertensive crisis**.

FOODS/BEVERAGES PATIENTS SHOULD AVOID
✓Cheese ✓Yogurt ✓Beer ✓Wine ✓Sauerkraut ✓Salami ✓Bologna ✓Liver ✓Chocolate ✓Coffee

NOTE: Anything that is fermented, aged, pickled, smoked or bacterially contaminated can be expected to contain a high amount of tyramine.

➲ MONITOR BLOOD PRESSURE FREQUENTLY ➲

DRUG-DRUG INTERACTIONS
Since MAOIs effectively enhance the activity of serotonin and norepinephrine, serious drug interactions can occur when they are combined with other medications that do the same thing. When combined with medications that enhance serotonin activity (e.g. selective serotonin reuptake inhibitors [SSRIs], serotonin-norepinephrine reuptake inhibitors [SNRIs], tricyclic antidepressants [TCAs], triptans), potentially deadly **serotonin syndrome** can occur. When combined with medications that enhance norepinephrine activity (e.g. amphetamines, ephedrine, dopamine, norepinephrine-dopamine reuptake inhibitors [NDRIs], SNRIs, TCAs), a **hypertensive crisis** can occur.

NOTE: MAOIs should not be taken within about two weeks* of other agents that inhibit the reuptake of serotonin, norepinephrine, and/or dopamine (e.g. SSRIs, SNRIs, TCAs, NDRIs).
*The specific timeframe varies based on the medication in question.

NOT A FIRST CHOICE *for* TREATMENT *of* DEPRESSION
Because of the potential to cause a hypertensive crisis when taken with certain commonly consumed foods and beverages, and because of the plethora of potentially deadly drug interactions, MAOIs are typically reserved for patients who have failed to respond to other less toxic antidepressants like SSRIs, SNRIs, NDRIs or TCAs.

THE RECURRING THEMES *of* ANTIDEPRESSANTS
#1 Expect a slow onset of action (2+ weeks).   **#2** Avoid abrupt discontinuation.
#3 Monitor patients for worsening of depression and suicidal thoughts and/or behaviors.
#4 Avoid driving until the effects are known.   **#5** Avoid alcoholic beverages.

HECKMAN'S
NURSING PHARMACOLOGY SIMPLIFIED

TRIPTANS

COMMON EXAMPLES
Imitrex® (sumatriptan)   Maxalt® (rizatriptan)   Zomig® (zolmitriptan)

Drug Name Stem: –triptan

Mechanism: Triptans activate certain serotonin receptors (5-HT$_{1B/1D}$) found in intracranial blood vessels and sensory neurons in the trigeminal system. This results in constriction of cranial blood vessels and inhibition of pro-inflammatory neuropeptide release.

Common Uses: Migraine headaches
NOTE: Triptans should **not** be used to prevent migraine headaches.

↻ REPEAT DOSING
MAY REPEAT DOSE AFTER TWO HOURS
If the migraine recurs or only partially resolves after the initial dose, another dose may be administered after two hours. Do not administer a second dose if the first dose was completely ineffective.

LIMIT THE USE *of* TRIPTANS
DUE TO RISK *of* MEDICATION OVERUSE HEADACHES
Triptan use should be limited to four days per month on average. The safety of more frequent use has not been established. Of particular interest, the use of acute migraine drugs (such as triptans, ergotamine, and/or opioids) for ≥ 10 days per month can lead to "medication overuse headaches."

CONSEQUENCES *of the* MECHANISM
Migraines are thought to be caused in part by dilated cranial blood vessels pressing on nearby nociceptors. Triptans constrict these blood vessels to relieve the pressure and pain. While this may eliminate or ameliorate a migraine, the benefit is not without risk.

↑ RISK *of* ISCHEMIC EVENTS	↑ BLOOD PRESSURE
Predictably, constriction of blood vessels can cause life-threatening cardiovascular events, such as a heart attack or stroke. Triptans should never be used in patients with a history of ischemic disease.	Triptan use can increase blood pressure significantly, even leading to hypertensive crisis in rare cases. Consequently, triptans should never be used in patients with uncontrolled hypertension.

OTHER PATIENT EDUCATION POINTS

USE CAUTION WHEN DRIVING: Common side effects of triptans include somnolence and dizziness. Consequently, patients who are taking a triptan should be advised to avoid driving or operating machinery until the effects are known.

WATCH *for* SEROTONIN SYNDROME: Serotonin syndrome can occur with the use of a single agent (e.g. a triptan); however, the risk increases with the use of multiple serotonin-enhancing agents such as selective serotonin reuptake inhibitors, serotonin-norepinephrine reuptake inhibitors, tricyclic antidepressants, triptans, and/or St. John's Wort.

HECKMAN'S
NURSING PHARMACOLOGY SIMPLIFIED

TYPICAL ANTIPSYCHOTICS

THE MOST COMMON EXAMPLES
Haldol® (haloperidol)   Thorazine® (chlorpromazine)

Mechanism: Haloperidol selectively antagonizes dopamine (D_2) receptors.

Common Uses: Psychosis, schizophrenia, Tourette's syndrome, acute agitation

EXTRAPYRAMIDAL SYMPTOMS
Antagonism of dopamine can cause extrapyramidal symptoms such as involuntary movements, slow/impaired voluntary movements, rigidity, tremor, restlessness, and **tardive dyskinesia**—a potentially irreversible and untreatable condition characterized by involuntary rhythmic movements (e.g. "lip-smacking"). Patients should report involuntary muscle movements to their healthcare provider immediately.

CONTRAINDICATIONS *for* TYPICAL ANTIPSYCHOTICS

PARKINSON'S DISEASE
Drug therapies for Parkinson's disease work by activating dopamine receptors in the central nervous system (CNS). Since typical antipsychotics work by antagonizing dopamine receptors, they can worsen the symptoms of Parkinson's disease.

SEVERE CNS DEPRESSION
Typical antipsychotics cause sedation. To avoid potentially deadly CNS/respiratory depression, comatose patients or patients on large doses of other CNS depressants (e.g. opioids, anesthesia, alcohol) should not receive typical antipsychotics.

OTHER SIDE EFFECTS *of* TYPICAL ANTIPSYCHOTICS
Besides dopamine, antipsychotics also interfere with the activity of several other neurotransmitters such as acetylcholine, catecholamines (e.g. epinephrine), and histamine, causing a variety of side effects.

ANTIADRENERGIC EFFECTS	ANTICHOLINERGIC EFFECTS*	ANTIHISTAMINE EFFECTS
Hypotension	Dry mouth, constipation	Sedation

See page 44 for a detailed list of anticholinergic effects.

NEUROLEPTIC MALIGNANT SYNDROME
Though rare, antipsychotics can cause neuroleptic malignant syndrome, a potentially life-threatening reaction characterized by high fever, sweating, tachycardia, irregular blood pressure, confusion, and muscle rigidity.

ANTIPSYCHOTICS LOWER THE SEIZURE THRESHOLD

PATIENTS SHOULD NOT DISCONTINUE ABRUPTLY AFTER LONG-TERM USE
Abrupt discontinuation of typical antipsychotics can lead to withdrawal symptoms resembling tardive dyskinesia. To discontinue haloperidol, gradual dose reduction is recommended.

HECKMAN'S
NURSING PHARMACOLOGY SIMPLIFIED

ATYPICAL ANTIPSYCHOTICS

COMMON EXAMPLES
Clozaril® (clozapine)   Risperdal® (risperidone)   Seroquel® (quetiapine)
Zyprexa® (olanzapine)   Geodon® (ziprasidone)   Abilify® (aripiprazole)

Mechanism: Atypical antidepressants antagonize dopamine (D_2) and serotonin ($5\text{-}HT_{2A}$) receptors.

Common Uses: Schizophrenia, bipolar disorder, irritability associated with autistic disorder

UNIQUE CHARACTERISTICS of ATYPICAL ANTIPSYCHOTICS

LOWER RISK of EXTRAPYRAMIDAL SYMPTOMS
The atypical antipsychotics are also known as second generation antipsychotics. They are "atypical" because they are generally less likely to cause extrapyramidal symptoms such as involuntary muscle movements, rigidity, restlessness, tremor and tardive dyskinesia.

HIGHER RISK of METABOLIC SIDE EFFECTS
Metabolic side effects including hyperglycemia, dyslipidemia, and weight gain are more likely with atypical antipsychotics. Depending on the situation, blood glucose, lipids, and body weight monitoring may be required at baseline and throughout treatment.

USE CAUTIOUSLY IN PATIENTS WITH PARKINSON'S DISEASE
Atypical antipsychotics are not contraindicated in patients with Parkinson's disease; however, since antipsychotics oppose dopamine, they may interfere with Parkinson's disease medications.

THE COMMON THEMES of ANTIPSYCHOTICS
Though there are some key differences, such as those outlined above, the typical and atypical antipsychotics have a lot in common. For example, nearly all of them are associated with:
✓ Extrapyramidal symptoms   ✓ Increased risk of seizures   ✓ Agranulocytosis
✓ Hypotension   ✓ Anticholinergic effects   ✓ Sedation
✓ Neuroleptic malignant syndrome

THE RELATIONSHIP BETWEEN DOPAMINE, PSYCHOSIS, and EXTRAPYRAMIDAL SYMPTOMS

Psychosis — EXCESSIVE DOPAMINE ACTIVITY ... LOW DOPAMINE ACTIVITY — Extrapyramidal Symptoms

AGRANULOCYTOSIS from CLOZARIL® (CLOZAPINE)
Of all the antipsychotics, clozapine has the greatest potential to cause life-threatening agranulocytosis. For this reason, routine blood work is required for any patient that uses clozapine. This includes monitoring of the patient's absolute neutrophil count as frequently as once per week.

NOTE: Clozapine is typically reserved for patients who fail to respond to other antipsychotics.

HECKMAN'S
NURSING PHARMACOLOGY SIMPLIFIED

PROKINETIC-ANTIEMETIC

THE MOST COMMON EXAMPLE
Reglan® (metoclopramide)

Mechanism: Metoclopramide antagonizes dopamine (D_2) receptors in the chemoreceptor trigger zone and stimulates upper gastrointestinal motility by sensitizing the tissue to the effects of acetylcholine.

Common Uses: Gastroesophageal reflux disease (GERD) that fails to respond to conventional therapies, diabetic gastroparesis, postoperative or chemotherapy-induced nausea/vomiting

---

THE 12-WEEK LIMIT
DUE TO RISK *of* TARDIVE DYSKINESIA

Like the antipsychotics, metoclopramide is a dopamine (D_2) receptor antagonist that carries a risk of extrapyramidal symptoms and tardive dyskinesia, an untreatable and potentially irreversible movement disorder. The risk of developing tardive dyskinesia increases with duration of treatment. To minimize the risk of tardive dyskinesia, metoclopramide should not be used for more than 12 weeks.

NOTE: Like the antipsychotics, metoclopramide may exacerbate symptoms of Parkinson's disease.

THE MOST COMMON SIDE EFFECTS *of* METOCLOPRAMIDE

#1 RESTLESSNESS	#2 DROWSINESS
Have patients stop taking metoclopramide and notify their healthcare provider immediately if they experience motor restlessness, as this may indicate the onset of extrapyramidal symptoms or tardive dyskinesia.	Tell patients to avoid driving or operating machinery until the effects are known. Also, avoid the use of other central nervous system depressants (e.g. opioids, benzodiazepines, alcohol) while taking metoclopramide.

DRUG INTERACTION
METOCLOPRAMIDE + ANTIPSYCHOTICS

Metoclopramide and antipsychotics should not be used concurrently due to the heightened risk of inducing extrapyramidal symptoms, tardive dyskinesia, and neuroleptic malignant syndrome.

THE 30 MINUTE RULE
for METOCLOPRAMIDE ADMINISTRATION

GERD *or* DIABETIC GASTROPARESIS	CHEMOTHERAPY-INDUCED NAUSEA/VOMITING
Administer **30 minutes** before meals and at bedtime.	Administer the initial dose **30 minutes** before chemotherapy.

REGLAN® (METOCLOPRAMIDE) LOWERS THE SEIZURE THRESHOLD

5-HT$_3$ RECEPTOR ANTAGONISTS

COMMON EXAMPLES
Zofran® (ondansetron)   Aloxi® (palonosetron)   Kytril® (granisetron)

Drug Name Stem: –setron

Mechanism: 5-HT$_3$ receptor antagonists block a subtype of serotonin receptors (5-HT$_3$) located centrally in the chemoreceptor trigger zone and peripherally in vagal neurons of the upper gastrointestinal tract, producing an antiemetic effect.

Common Uses: Nausea/vomiting

ANTIEMETIC

THE MOST NOTABLE SIDE EFFECTS

HEADACHE and CONSTIPATION
The most common side effects associated with 5-HT$_3$ receptor antagonists are headache and constipation.

RISK of CARDIAC ARRHYTHMIAS
Particularly applies to patients with electrolyte abnormalities, heart failure, bradyarrhythmias, and those taking other medications that can prolong the QT interval.

RISK of SEROTONIN SYNDROME
Can occur with the use of a single agent; however, the risk increases with the use of multiple serotonin-enhancing agents, such as SSRIs, SNRIs, TCAs, triptans, and/or St. John's Wort.

Abbreviations: SSRIs, selective serotonin reuptake inhibitors; SNRIs, serotonin-norepinephrine reuptake inhibitors; TCAs, tricyclic antidepressants.

NOTE: Compared to other antiemetics, they are generally well-tolerated with few side effects.

ZOFRAN® ORALLY DISINTEGRATING TABLET (ODT)
With dry hands, place the ODT on top of the tongue, allow to dissolve, then swallow with saliva.

NOTE: Designed to dissolve quickly in saliva without administration of water.

THE 30-MINUTE RULE
for PREVENTING CHEMOTHERAPY-INDUCED NAUSEA/VOMITING
5-HT$_3$ receptor antagonists are commonly used for the prevention of chemotherapy-induced nausea and vomiting. The key word is **prevention**. To get the best possible result, it is crucial to administer the first dose about 30 minutes before the start of chemotherapy.

HECKMAN'S
NURSING PHARMACOLOGY SIMPLIFIED

LAXATIVES

Bulk-Forming Laxatives
Metamucil® (psyllium fiber)
Citrucel® (methylcellulose)
FiberCon® (polycarbophil)
Mechanism: Fiber absorbs water and swells up, exerting pressure on the intestinal wall, which triggers peristalsis.

Osmotic Laxatives
MiraLAX® (polyethylene glycol 3350)
Milk of Magnesia (magnesium hydroxide)
Generlac® (lactulose)
Mechanism: Osmotic laxatives draw water into the intestinal lumen, which increases water content in the stool, producing a laxative effect.

Stimulant Laxatives
Senokot® (sennosides)   Dulcolax® (bisacodyl)
Mechanism: Sennosides and bisacodyl irritate the intestinal mucosa, producing large contractions in the colon (large intestine).

Stool Softeners
Colace® (docusate)
Mechanism: Docusate, a surfactant, facilitates the incorporation of water and fat, ultimately softening and increasing the mass of the stool.

TIME TO PRODUCE BOWEL MOVEMENT BASED ON ROUTE *of* ADMINISTRATION
Rectal Enema > Rectal Suppository > Oral Formulation

TIME TO PRODUCE BOWEL MOVEMENT (BM) BASED ON ACTIVE INGREDIENT

magnesium hydroxide	½ – 6 hours
sennosides, bisacodyl*	6 – 12 hours
lactulose	1 – 2 days
psyllium fiber, methylcellulose, polycarbophil, polyethylene glycol, docusate	1 – 3 days

*__EXCEPTIONS:__ Suppository produces a BM in under 60 minutes, and enema produces a BM in under 20 minutes.

ADVISE PATIENTS TO DRINK PLENTY *of* FLUIDS
Constipation is exacerbated and may even be caused by a lack of adequate hydration. Also, most laxatives rely on water to exert their effect. So, patients who are constipated should be advised to drink plenty of fluids.

MOST COMMON SIDE EFFECTS
Minor bloating, abdominal cramping, and flatulence (bulk-forming and osmotic laxatives)
Abdominal pain and cramping, diarrhea, nausea/vomiting (stimulant laxatives)
Abdominal cramping and diarrhea (stool softeners)

DRUGS INTERACTIONS WITH BULK-FORMING LAXATIVES
The fiber in bulk-forming laxatives can bind and deactivate many medications. To avoid interactions, administer bulk-forming laxatives at least two hours before or two hours after other medications.

ANTIDIARRHEALS

COMMON EXAMPLES
Imodium® (loperamide)   Lomotil® (diphenoxylate/atropine)

Mechanism: Loperamide and diphenoxylate stimulate opioid receptors in the gut wall, reducing peristalsis and slowing intestinal motility.

Common Uses: Diarrhea

IMODIUM® (LOPERAMIDE)
OTC
Imodium® is a non-controlled substance that is available over-the-counter without a prescription.

LOMOTIL® (DIPHENOXYLATE/ATROPINE)
C-V
Lomotil® is a Schedule V controlled substance that is only available with a prescription.

REPLENISH FLUID and ELECTROLYTES
While antidiarrheals may be helpful for treating diarrhea in some patients, it is important to remember that diarrhea causes a loss of fluid and electrolytes that must be replenished to prevent dehydration.

CAPITALIZING ON OPIOID-INDUCED CONSTIPATION
Constipation is the most common side effect of opioids. While other opioid side effects tend to diminish as tolerance develops, opioid-induced constipation does not improve with continued use. Opioid-induced constipation occurs when opioids bind to and activate opiate receptors in the gut wall, resulting in decreased intestinal motility. Drug manufacturers capitalize on this side effect with drugs like loperamide and diphenoxylate for the treatment of diarrhea.

THE ROLE of ATROPINE IN LOMOTIL®
Lomotil® contains atropine, not for any therapeutic effect, but as an abuse deterrent. This is necessary because diphenoxylate is a controlled substance. If a person attempts to abuse the diphenoxylate content by taking excessive doses of Lomotil®, the relatively large dose of atropine they receive as a consequence triggers an unpleasant experience of nausea/vomiting.

COMMON SIDE EFFECTS
✓Constipation ✓Nausea/Vomiting ✓Drowsiness
NOTE: Common side effects of antidiarrheals are similar to those of opioid analgesics.

HECKMAN'S
NURSING PHARMACOLOGY SIMPLIFIED

ANTACIDS

COMMON EXAMPLES
Tums® (calcium carbonate)   Rolaids® (calcium carbonate/magnesium hydroxide)
Maalox® Advanced (aluminum hydroxide/magnesium hydroxide/simethicone)
Gaviscon® (aluminum hydroxide/magnesium carbonate)

Mechanism: Antacids work by chemically neutralizing gastric acid (hydrochloric acid).

Common Uses: Dyspepsia

IMMEDIATE RESULTS
While antacids may not be as effective as H2 blockers or proton pump inhibitors, they do have a quicker onset of action.

EFFECT *of* ANTACIDS ON GASTROINTESTINAL (GI) MOTILITY
Constipation: Calcium (Ca^{2+}), Aluminum (Al^{3+})   Diarrhea: Magnesium (Mg^{2+})

Many antacids combine magnesium with calcium or aluminum to have a balanced effect on GI motility. With these combination products, most patients don't experience constipation or diarrhea.

BELCHING, BLOATING, *and* FLATULENCE
Calcium carbonate is unique. The reaction between calcium carbonate ($CaCO_3$) and hydrochloric acid (HCl) yields water (H_2O), carbon dioxide (CO_2), and calcium chloride ($CaCl_2$).

$$CaCO_3 + HCl \Rightarrow H_2O + CO_2 + CaCl_2$$

Acid neutralized. Mission accomplished, right? Yes, but not without consequences. As we know, carbon dioxide is a gas. So, the most common side effects of calcium carbonate are exactly what you would expect—belching, bloating, and flatulence.

DRUG INTERACTIONS
Most of the drug interactions involve chelation of polyvalent cations (e.g. calcium, magnesium, aluminum). Other drug interactions result from reduced gastric and urinary acidity. Generally, interactions can be avoided by separating administration from other drugs by at least two hours.

SIMETHICONE
Simethicone is a surface-active agent (or "surfactant") similar to a detergent. It breaks the surface tension on gas bubbles in the GI tract, providing relief from bloating, gas pains, and flatulence.

PROTON PUMP INHIBITORS

COMMON EXAMPLES
Prilosec® (omeprazole)   Nexium® (esomeprazole)   Protonix® (pantoprazole)
Prevacid® (lansoprazole)   Dexilant® (dexlansoprazole)

Drug Name Stem: –prazole

Mechanism: Proton pump inhibitors (PPIs) block hydrogen-potassium ATPase (the "proton pump") in gastric parietal cells, ultimately reducing stomach acid production.

Common Uses: Gastric ulcers, duodenal ulcers, stress ulcer prophylaxis, *H. pylori* infection, erosive esophagitis, gastroesophageal reflux disease (GERD), dyspepsia

---

TAKE BEFORE A MEAL *for* BEST RESULTS
PPIs must be introduced into an acidic environment to be activated. Ingestion of food stimulates gastric acid production. For this reason, PPIs generally work best when taken before a meal.

80–95%
REDUCTION IN STOMACH ACID PRODUCTION
Proton pump inhibitors reduce stomach acid production by approximately 80–95%, making them among the most potent acid reducers available.

INCREASED RISK *of* CLOSTRIDIUM DIFFICILE-ASSOCIATED DIARRHEA
When used concurrently with antibiotics, the use of a PPI increases the risk of *C. difficile* infection. This makes sense when you think of stomach acid in the context of a defense mechanism. The acid kills bacteria and other pathogens in the GI tract. Less stomach acid production means less killing of GI bacteria, which opens the door to the type of bacterial overgrowth seen in *C. difficile* infection.

DRAWBACKS *of* LONG-TERM TREATMENT
Short-term proton pump inhibitor use is associated with a few mild side effects (e.g. headache, abdominal pain, nausea/vomiting, diarrhea), but chronic suppression of stomach acid production can increase the risk of deficiencies in vitamins and minerals that rely on stomach acid for optimal absorption.

3+ MONTHS *of* TREATMENT	12+ MONTHS *of* TREATMENT	36+ MONTHS *of* TREATMENT
MAGNESIUM DEFICIENCY	OSTEOPOROSIS/BONE FRACTURES	VITAMIN B_{12} DEFICIENCY

OVER-THE-COUNTER AVAILABILITY
Prilosec OTC® (omeprazole 20 mg), Nexium® 24 HR (esomeprazole 20 mg), and Prevacid® 24 HR (lansoprazole 15 mg) are each available over-the-counter. Dexilant® (dexlansoprazole), Protonix (pantoprazole), and higher strengths of the other PPIs are available by prescription only. Due to the potential for long-term side effects, patients should not use over-the-counter PPIs for more than 14 days without consulting a healthcare provider.

HECKMAN'S
NURSING PHARMACOLOGY SIMPLIFIED

H2 RECEPTOR ANTAGONISTS

COMMON EXAMPLES
Zantac® (ranitidine)   Pepcid® (famotidine)   Tagamet® (cimetidine)

Drug Name Stem: –tidine

Mechanism: H2 receptor antagonists ("H2 blockers") block H2 receptors, which are predominantly located on parietal cells in the stomach, ultimately reducing histamine-mediated stomach acid production.

Common Uses: Gastric ulcers, duodenal ulcers, stress ulcer prophylaxis, erosive esophagitis, gastroesophageal reflux disease (GERD), dyspepsia

ONSET of ACTION
With an onset of action occurring within 60 minutes of administration,
H2 blockers begin working faster than proton pump inhibitors (PPIs).

70%
REDUCTION IN STOMACH ACID PRODUCTION
H2 blockers reduce stomach acid production by approximately 70 percent, meaning they are less effective at suppressing acid production compared to PPIs.

INCREASED RISK of CLOSTRIDIUM DIFFICILE-ASSOCIATED DIARRHEA
Particularly when used with antibiotics, the use of an H2 blocker increases the risk of *C. difficile* infection. This makes sense when you think of stomach acid in the context of a defense mechanism. The acid kills bacteria and other pathogens in the gastrointestinal (GI) tract. Less stomach acid production means less killing of GI bacteria, which opens the door to the type of bacterial overgrowth seen in *C. difficile* infection.

CIMETIDINE-INDUCED GYNECOMASTIA
Gynecomastia is a condition characterized by enlarged breast tissue in boys and men. Although rare, Tagamet® (cimetidine) is notorious for causing drug-induced gynecomastia.

OVER-THE-COUNTER AVAILABILITY
Zantac® (ranitidine 75 mg & 150 mg), Pepcid® AC (famotidine 10 & 20 mg), Tagamet® (cimetidine 200 mg), and Axid® AR (nizatidine 75 mg) are available over-the-counter. Higher strengths are available by prescription only. As with PPIs, patients should not use over-the-counter H2 blockers for more than 14 days without consulting a healthcare provider.

HECKMAN'S
NURSING PHARMACOLOGY SIMPLIFIED

GASTROINTESTINAL PROTECTANTS

THE MOST COMMON EXAMPLE
Carafate® (sucralfate)

Mechanism: Sucralfate forms a protective coating over the interior of the stomach and inhibits pepsin.

Common Uses: Duodenal ulcers

GENERALLY WELL-TOLERATED

LOCAL ACTION
Carafate® (sucralfate) is given by mouth and works locally, rather than systemically, by coating the lining of the stomach and inhibiting pepsin, an enzyme that breaks down proteins.

MINIMAL ABSORPTION
Carafate® (sucralfate) is minimally absorbed from the gastrointestinal tract, and adheres particularly well to damaged tissue, such as ulcers.

FEW SIDE EFFECTS
Because Carafate® (sucralfate) is minimally absorbed, there are few side effects. The most common side effect is constipation, which only occurs in about 2% of patients.

MANY DRUG INTERACTIONS

ADMINISTER WITHOUT FOOD
Administer Carafate® (sucralfate) on an empty stomach at least one hour before or two hours after a meal. If administered with food, sucralfate will bind to the food rather than to the lining of the stomach.

SEPARATE OTHER MEDICATIONS
Carafate® (sucralfate) interferes with the absorption of several medications. Avoid drug interactions by administering any other medication(s) at least two hours before administering sucralfate.

ORAL SUSPENSION: SHAKE WELL
The liquid form of Carafate® (sucralfate) is a suspension. The active ingredient will settle to the bottom over time. For this reason, it is important to remember to shake the liquid suspension well prior to measuring and administering the dose to the patient.

HECKMAN'S
NURSING PHARMACOLOGY SIMPLIFIED
PROSTAGLANDIN ANALOGS

THE MOST COMMON EXAMPLE
Cytotec® (misoprostol)

Mechanism: Misoprostol, a synthetic prostaglandin E1 analog, inhibits gastric acid secretion and stimulates gastric mucus secretion. Misoprostol also stimulates uterine contractions.

Common Uses: Prevention of non-steroidal anti-inflammatory drug (NSAID)-induced gastric ulcers, induction of cervical ripening, termination of pregnancy

ROUTE of ADMINISTRATION
Misoprostol tablets should be given orally for every indication except cervical ripening. When used for cervical ripening, administer vaginally.

MISOPROSTOL + NSAIDs
Prostaglandins stimulate gastric mucus secretion. Meanwhile, NSAIDs inhibit prostaglandin synthesis. In the presence of NSAID use, prostaglandin-mediated mucus production is reduced, leaving the lining of the stomach exposed to the corrosive effects of gastric acid.

ABORTIFACIENT
Being a prostaglandin analog, misoprostol can stimulate uterine contractions. For this reason, the use of misoprostol can result in abortion, premature birth, and uterine rupture. It is used in combination with mifepristone (RU-486) or methotrexate to terminate pregnancies.

PREGNANCY CATEGORY X
Misoprostol has teratogenic and abortifacient properties, and pregnant women should never use it to prevent NSAID-induced gastric ulcers.

REMIND PATIENTS NEVER TO SHARE PRESCRIPTION MEDICATIONS WITH OTHERS

MOST COMMON SIDE EFFECTS
#1 Diarrhea*
#2 Abdominal pain/cramps

These side effects are logical considering the pharmacologic effects of misoprostol include stimulation of gastric mucus production and stimulation of uterine contractions.

*To reduce the incidence of diarrhea, misoprostol should be administered after meals and at bedtime.

HECKMAN'S
NURSING PHARMACOLOGY SIMPLIFIED

INSULIN

Mealtime Insulin	Rapid Acting	Apidra®, Humalog®, NovoLog®	Available Rx only
	Short-Acting	Humulin R®, Novolin R®	Available OTC
Basal Insulin	Intermediate Acting	Humulin N®, Novolin N®	
	Long Acting	Lantus®, Levemir®, Toujeo®, Tresiba®	Available Rx only
NOTE: Humulin® R U-500 insulin is 5× more concentrated than standard U-100 insulin. Always inject U-500 insulin with a U-500 syringe to reduce the risk of potentially fatal inadvertent overdose.			

Mechanism: Insulin stimulates cellular uptake of glucose from the bloodstream.
Common Uses: Type 1 and type 2 diabetes mellitus

HYPOGLYCEMIA: THE #1 SIDE EFFECT *of* INSULIN
Monitor blood glucose and watch for signs/symptoms of hypoglycemia (e.g. tremor, tachycardia, and sweating).

DO NOT SHAKE INSULIN
Humulin® N and Novolin® N (insulin NPH) have a cloudy appearance and must be gently rotated prior to use. All other forms of insulin are clear and do not require gentle mixing prior to use. In any case, never shake insulin vigorously, as this can denature and deactivate the product.

NEVER USE ONE PEN *for* MULTIPLE PATIENTS
Even when the needle is changed, there is still a risk of transmitting bloodborne pathogens when an injection pen is shared between patients.

DO NOT COMBINE MULTIPLE INSULIN FORMULATIONS IN THE SAME SYRINGE
The activity of the insulin may be altered when different insulin formulations are drawn up in the same syringe.
EXCEPTION: Insulin NPH (Humulin N® or Novolin N®) can be combined in the same syringe with regular human insulin (Humulin R® or Novolin R®), provided the regular human insulin is drawn up first, and the injection is administered immediately after adding insulin NPH to the syringe.

ADMINISTER INSULIN BY SUBCUTANEOUS INJECTION
NOTE: Under medical supervision, rapid or short-acting insulin may be administered intravenously.

REFRIGERATE UNOPENED INSULIN VIALS *and* PENS
Insulin is stable until the expiration date printed on the label only when stored unopened under refrigeration. Once opened and/or when stored at room temperature, most insulin is stable for about one month; however, the exact amount of time varies between products. See below for select examples.

	NovoLog®	Novolin® R	Novolin® N	Lantus®	Levemir®	Tresiba®
Vial	28 days	42 days	42 days	28 days	42 days	N/A
Pen	28 days	28 days	14 days	28 days	42 days	56 days

NOTE: Do not freeze insulin. Discard if frozen.

THE ANTIDOTE *for* INSULIN
GlucaGen® (glucagon), a hormone that stimulates the conversion of glycogen to glucose.

HECKMAN'S
NURSING PHARMACOLOGY SIMPLIFIED

BIGUANIDES

THE ONLY EXAMPLE COMMERCIALLY AVAILABLE IN THE UNITED STATES
Glucophage® (metformin)

Mechanism: Metformin decreases intestinal absorption of glucose, decreases the amount of glucose produced by the liver, and increases insulin sensitivity.

Common Uses: Type 2 diabetes mellitus

THE FIRST WEEK of TREATMENT

The most common side effect of metformin is diarrhea. This and other gastrointestinal (GI) side effects (e.g. nausea/vomiting, flatulence, indigestion) typically occur **during the first week** of treatment and then resolve spontaneously with continued use. The most common strategies for reducing the incidence of GI side effects:

1) Start at a low dose and increase gradually.
2) Use an extended-release formulation.

THE ADVANTAGES of EXTENDED-RELEASE METFORMIN

1) Reduced incidence of GI side effects compared to regular-release metformin.

	Glucophage® (metformin)	Glucophage® XR (metformin extended-release)
Diarrhea	53.2% of patients	9.6% of patients
Nausea/Vomiting	25.5% of patients	6.5% of patients

Data Source: Glucophage [package insert]. Princeton, NJ: Bristol-Myers Squibb Company; 2017.

2) Virtually odorless compared to regular-release metformin, which possesses a strong fish-like odor.

NOTE: Despite the advantages, extended-release metformin tends to be considerably more expensive.

ADMINISTER WITH A MEAL

Metformin does not stimulate insulin secretion and is consequently unlikely to cause hypoglycemia. Unlike sulfonylureas, administration of metformin with a meal is not a strategy to prevent hypoglycemia, but rather a strategy to reduce the incidence of GI side effects like diarrhea and nausea/vomiting.

LACTIC ACIDOSIS

Metformin is associated with lactic acidosis, a rare but potentially fatal condition that is more likely to occur in patients with renal impairment. Administration of iodinated contrast media can trigger an acute decline in renal function, further increasing the risk of lactic acidosis in patients taking metformin. For this reason, it is common for metformin to be discontinued temporarily in patients receiving iodinated contrast agents.

VITAMIN B_{12} DEFICIENCY

Long-term use of metformin can lead to vitamin B_{12} deficiency and pernicious anemia. Vitamin B_{12} supplementation (e.g. monthly intramuscular injections of cyanocobalamin 1,000 mcg) may be necessary.

**HECKMAN'S
NURSING PHARMACOLOGY SIMPLIFIED**

ORAL HYPOGLYCEMIC AGENTS

ALL ORAL HYPOGLYCEMICS ARE APPROVED ONLY *for the* TREATMENT *of* TYPE 2 DIABETES MELLITUS

SULFONYLUREAS
DiaBeta® (glyburide)   Amaryl® (glimepiride)   Glucotrol® (glipizide)
Mechanism: Sulfonylureas lower blood glucose by stimulating insulin release from the pancreas.

RISK *of* HYPOGLYCEMIA
All sulfonylureas can cause hypoglycemia, but the risk is greater with glyburide due to its relatively long elimination rate.

SULFA ALLERGY
Sulfonylureas have a sulfonamide component that can trigger an allergic reaction in patients with a sulfonamide (or "sulfa") allergy.

➲ Administer with a meal ☙

THIAZOLIDINEDIONES
Actos® (pioglitazone)   Avandia® (rosiglitazone)
Drug Name Stem: –glitazone
Mechanism: Thiazolidinediones activate PPARγ. This enhances insulin sensitivity, making cells more responsive to insulin.

HEART FAILURE
Thiazolidinediones may cause or exacerbate heart failure and are contraindicated in patients with moderate–severe heart failure.

DPP-4 INHIBITORS
Tradjenta® (linagliptin)   Januvia® (sitagliptin)
Drug Name Stem: –gliptin
Mechanism: DPP-4 inhibitors slow the breakdown of incretin, increasing insulin release in the presence of elevated glucose and decreasing glucagon release.

PANCREATITIS
DPP-4 inhibitors are associated with an increased risk of pancreatitis (rare). Look for persistent severe abdominal pain ± vomiting.

➲ Administer without regard to meals ☙

SGLT-2 INHIBITORS
Invokana® (canagliflozin)   Farxiga® (dapagliflozin)   Jardiance® (empagliflozin)
Drug Name Stem: –agliflozin
Mechanism: Sodium-glucose co-transporter 2 (SGLT-2) inhibitors block glucose reabsorption, effectively lowering the renal threshold for glucose and increasing the amount of glucose leaving the body via the urine.

RENAL SIDE EFFECTS
Directly related to the mechanism of action (increased urinary excretion of glucose), SGLT-2 inhibitors can cause urinary tract infections, genital yeast infections, increased urination, and impaired renal function.

➲ Administer in the morning with or without food ☙

LINKING MECHANISM TO ADMINISTRATION INSTRUCTIONS
Sulfonylureas directly stimulate insulin secretion, so they must be taken with a meal to prevent hypoglycemia. Thiazolidinediones, DPP-4 inhibitors, and SGLT-2 inhibitors do not directly stimulate insulin secretion and are consequently unlikely to cause hypoglycemia.

GLP-1 AGONISTS

COMMON EXAMPLES
Byetta®, Bydureon® (exenatide)   Victoza® (liraglutide)   Trulicity® (dulaglutide)

Mechanism: Glucagon-like peptide-1 (GLP-1) agonists mimic incretin, which increases insulin release in the presence of elevated glucose levels, decreases glucagon release, and delays gastric emptying.

Common Uses: Type 2 diabetes mellitus

ROUTE of ADMINISTRATION
GLP-1 agonists are peptides (short-chain amino acids). The digestive tract indiscriminately breaks them down for digestion; however, for these medications to exert the intended pharmacologic effect, they must maintain their chemical structure, which means they cannot be administered orally. They must be injected.

ADMINISTER GLP-1 AGONISTS BY SUBCUTANEOUS INJECTION ONLY

NEVER USE ONE PEN for MULTIPLE PATIENTS
Even when the needle is changed, there is still a risk of transmitting bloodborne pathogens when an injection pen is shared between patients.

THE #1 SIDE EFFECT: NAUSEA
GLP-1 agonists delay gastric emptying, which produces a feeling of fullness. It should be no surprise that these medications can cause some patients to feel nauseous. Nausea is particularly common at the start of treatment and usually resolves with continued use.

PANCREATITIS
Like DPP-4 inhibitors, which also work by enhancing incretin activity, GLP-1 agonists can cause acute pancreatitis, the hallmark symptom of which is severe abdominal pain ± vomiting. Report these symptoms to the physician.

THYROID C-CELL TUMORS
GLP-1 agonists cause thyroid C-cell tumors in rats. The risk in humans is unknown. Report symptoms of thyroid tumor (e.g. a lump in the neck, pain or difficulty swallowing or breathing, persistent hoarseness) to the physician.

BENEFIT OVER DPP-4 INHIBITORS
GLP-1 agonists delay gastric emptying; whereas DPP-4 inhibitors do not. Delayed gastric emptying produces a feeling of fullness that may help patients to eat less and lose weight. Since weight-loss can reverse type 2 diabetes mellitus in certain patients, this is a substantial benefit over DPP-4 inhibitors.

STORE IN THE REFRIGERATOR
GLP-1 agonists are stable until the expiration date printed on the label only when stored unopened under refrigeration. Once opened and/or when stored at room temperature, GLP-1 agonists are stable for about one month; however, the exact amount of time varies between products. See below.

Byetta®	Bydureon®	Victoza®	Trulicity®
30 days	28 days	30 days	14 days

NOTE: Do not freeze GLP-1 agonists. Discard if frozen.

HECKMAN'S
NURSING PHARMACOLOGY SIMPLIFIED

SYNTHETIC THYROID HORMONE

COMMON EXAMPLES
Synthroid®, Levoxyl® (levothyroxine)

Mechanism: Levothyroxine mimics thyroxine (T4), a hormone that primarily regulates metabolism.

Common Uses: Hypothyroidism

ADJUST DOSE BASED ON THYROID STIMULATING HORMONE (TSH) LEVELS*
The pituitary gland releases TSH to trigger secretion of additional T4 from the thyroid gland. Consequently, a low TSH level indicates an abundance of T4, and a high TSH level indicates a lack of T4. If TSH is low, then decrease the dose. If TSH is high, increase the dose.

*Assuming the diagnosis is primary hypothyroidism. In cases of secondary or tertiary hypothyroidism (rare), dosing is based on serum free T4 levels. In these cases, if free T4 is low then increase dose, and vice versa.

LEVOTHYROXINE REQUIRES 4–6 WEEKS TO REACH PEAK THERAPEUTIC EFFECT

SYMPTOMS OF HYPOTHYROIDISM	SYMPTOMS OF HYPERTHYROIDISM
Bradycardia, Constipation, Cold Intolerance, Fatigue/Somnolence, Weight Gain	Tachycardia, Diarrhea, Heat Intolerance, Anxiety/Insomnia, Weight Loss

NOTE: Excessive doses of levothyroxine can produce symptoms identical to hyperthyroidism.

COLOR-CODED TABLETS
Levothyroxine tablet color is standardized based on strength.
For example, 100 mcg tablets are always yellow, regardless of the brand or manufacturer.

TAKE ON AN EMPTY STOMACH
Levothyroxine absorption is negatively impacted by various foods, medications, and supplements. For optimal absorption, instruct patients to take levothyroxine on an empty stomach about 30–60 minutes before breakfast.

SEPARATE BY AT LEAST FOUR HOURS
Calcium and **iron** bind to and deactivate levothyroxine. **Antacids** neutralize acid needed to absorb levothyroxine. To avoid these interactions, separate levothyroxine from calcium, iron, and/or antacids by at least four hours.

DO NOT MIX LEVOTHYROXINE INJECTION WITH OTHER INTRAVENOUS FLUIDS

MONITOR BLOOD GLUCOSE CLOSELY IN PATIENTS WITH DIABETES
Starting, stopping, or changing the dose of levothyroxine inevitably affects metabolism and blood glucose.

NOT A WEIGHT-LOSS AGENT
The use of thyroid hormones by patients with normal thyroid function is unlikely to cause weight-loss and could trigger life-threatening cardiac symptoms (e.g. tachycardia, hypertension, angina pectoris, cardiac arrhythmias).

HECKMAN'S
NURSING PHARMACOLOGY SIMPLIFIED

ANTITHYROID DRUGS

COMMON EXAMPLES
Propacil® (propylthiouracil)   Tapazole® (methimazole)

Mechanism: Propylthiouracil (PTU) and methimazole (MMI) inhibit thyroid hormone synthesis.

Common Uses: Hyperthyroidism

PTU
PROPYLTHIOURACIL
PTU has a higher risk of liver toxicity.

1ST TRIMESTER DRUG OF CHOICE
Since MMI carries a higher risk of birth defects in the first trimester of pregnancy, PTU is the first trimester drug of choice.

MMI
METHIMAZOLE
MMI has a higher risk of birth defects.

2ND/3RD TRIMESTER DRUG OF CHOICE
Since the risk of MMI-related birth defects decreases after the first trimester, MMI is the second and third trimester drug of choice.

MEDICATION-INDUCED
HYPOTHYROIDISM
Antithyroid drugs interfere with thyroid hormone production; however, too much interference can lead to hypothyroidism. For this reason, thyroid stimulating hormone and free thyroxine (T4) levels should be monitored and drug doses should be adjusted accordingly.

SERIOUS ADVERSE REACTIONS

LIVER TOXICITY
Patients on PTU or MMI should notify their healthcare provider immediately if they develop symptoms of liver dysfunction such as right upper quadrant pain, anorexia, and pruritus.

AGRANULOCYTOSIS
Patients on PTU or MMI should notify their healthcare provider immediately if they develop symptoms of agranulocytosis such as fever and sore throat.

THE #1 SIDE EFFECT: SKIN RASH
Skin rash is the most common side effect of antithyroid drugs (PTU and MMI). These rashes are usually mild and resolve spontaneously with continued treatment.

A REVIEW *of* TREATMENT OPTIONS *for* HYPERTHYROIDISM
There are three options for treating hyperthyroidism: antithyroid drugs, radioactive iodine, and surgical thyroidectomy. Antithyroid drugs are the only non-radioactive and non-surgical option.

**HECKMAN'S
NURSING PHARMACOLOGY SIMPLIFIED**

ANDROGENS

COMMON EXAMPLES
Depo® Testosterone (testosterone intramuscular injection)   Androgel® (testosterone topical gel)
Androderm® (testosterone transdermal patch)   Axiron® (testosterone topical solution)

Mechanism: Administration of pharmaceutical testosterone increases the amount of testosterone in the body, producing multiple androgenic effects.

Common Uses: Testosterone deficiency

ROUTES of ADMINISTRATION
After testosterone is absorbed from the gastrointestinal (GI) tract, it is quickly metabolized and deactivated by the liver. To solve this problem, all testosterone formulations are designed to enter the body by routes that avoid the GI tract. Most common routes are topical application and intramuscular injection.

IM

INTRAMUSCULAR INJECTION SITE
When administered by injection, testosterone should be injected **deeply into the gluteal muscle**. Never administer intravenously (IV).

C-III

CONTROLLED SUBSTANCE
Due to **potential for abuse** as an anabolic steroid (e.g. performance enhancement), testosterone is federally recognized as a Schedule III controlled substance.

X

PREGNANCY CATEGORY X
Testosterone is contraindicated in pregnant women.
Pregnant women should avoid skin contact with topical testosterone application sites in men.

↑ BLOOD CLOT RISK
Testosterone increases hematocrit levels (i.e. red blood cell count) and is associated with an increased risk of deep vein thrombosis, pulmonary embolism, myocardial infarction, and stroke.

↑ CANCER RISK
Long-term high-dose testosterone use is associate with an increased risk of liver cancer. Furthermore, testosterone is contraindicated in men with breast cancer (rare) or prostate cancer.

↓ BLOOD GLUCOSE IN PATIENTS WITH DIABETES
Testosterone can lower blood sugar in patients with diabetes.

SHAKE THE VIAL TO DISSOLVE CRYSTALS
As with all injections, visually inspect for particles and discoloration before administering. If crystals appear in testosterone injection liquid, then shake and warm the vial to dissolve the crystals prior to administration.

5-ALPHA-REDUCTASE INHIBITORS

COMMON EXAMPLES
Proscar®, Propecia® (finasteride)   Avodart® (dutasteride)

Drug Name Stem: –asteride

Mechanism: 5-alpha-reductase inhibitors block the enzyme (5-alpha-reductase) that converts testosterone to 5-dihydrotestosterone, a more powerful androgen that enlarges the prostate gland.

Common Uses: Benign prostatic hyperplasia (BPH), androgenic alopecia (male-pattern baldness)

THE MOST COMMON SIDE EFFECTS *of* 5-ALPHA REDUCTASE INHIBITORS

✓ Impotence   ✓ Decreased Libido   ✓ Decreased Ejaculate Volume   ✓ Gynecomastia

NOTE: Given that 5-dihydrotestosterone is more powerful than testosterone and that these medications effectively reduce the amount of 5-dihydrotestosterone in the body, these side effects are logical.

THE MOST SERIOUS SIDE EFFECT *of* 5-ALPHA-REDUCTASE INHIBITORS

✓ Increased Risk of High-Grade Prostate Cancer

A four-year and seven-year study involving the use of a 5-alpha-reductase inhibitor versus placebo revealed a 0.5% and 0.7% increase in the probability (respectively) of developing high-grade prostate cancer.

PREGNANCY CATEGORY X
The hormone 5-dihydrotestosterone is required for development of genitalia in the male fetus. Consequently, if a male fetus is exposed to a 5-alpha-reductase inhibitor, then the male sex organs may develop abnormally.

NOTE: There is no FDA-approved use for 5-alpha-reductase inhibitors in women.

WARNING *for* PREGNANT WOMEN
DO NOT HANDLE BROKEN TABLETS *or* LEAKING CAPSULES
Women who are pregnant or may become pregnant should not handle finasteride tablets that are broken or crushed or dutasteride capsules that are leaking. These medications can be absorbed through the skin and cause harm to the developing fetus.

NOTE: The outer shells of the tablet (finasteride) and capsule (dutasteride) do not contain active ingredients.

HECKMAN'S
NURSING PHARMACOLOGY SIMPLIFIED

COMBINATION HORMONE CONTRACEPTIVES

SELECT EXAMPLES
Ortho Cyclen® (norgestimate/ethinyl estradiol tablets)
Ortho Evra® (norelgestromin/ethinyl estradiol transdermal patch)
NuvaRing® (etonogestrel/ethinyl estradiol intravaginal ring)

Mechanism: The estrogens and progestins in combination hormone contraceptives inhibit ovulation, alter the endometrium, and thicken cervical mucus.

Common Uses: Prevention of pregnancy, treatment of acne

↑ BLOOD CLOT RISK
Combination hormone contraceptives are associated with an increased risk of cardiovascular events like heart attack or stroke. This risk is higher in cigarette smokers and women over the age of 35. Consequently, smokers over age 35 should **not** use combination hormone contraceptives.

[Age >35] + [Smoke Cigarettes] + [Combination Hormone Contraceptive] = High Risk of Blood Clot!

↑ CANCER RISK
Combination hormone contraceptives are contraindicated in patients with a history of breast cancer, endometrial cancer, or any other potentially estrogen-dependent cancers.

↓ EFFECT WITH ANTIBIOTICS
Antibiotics can reduce the effect of combination hormone contraceptives. A reduced effect is most likely when combination hormone contraceptives are taken with tetracycline or ampicillin.

PREGNANCY CATEGORY X
Combination hormone contraceptives are contraindicated in pregnant women.

MOST COMMON SIDE EFFECTS
#1 Breast Tenderness   #2 Nausea

A VARIETY OF CONVENIENT DOSAGE FORMS
Oral contraceptives ("birth control pills") are over 99% effective with perfect use; however, with typical use they are less effective (e.g. about 90–95% effective). That is to say, the typical patient is late or misses a dose on occasion, which reduces the contraceptive effect and increases the risk of unintended pregnancy. To reduce the chance of missing a dose, a variety of convenient dosage forms are available.

Oral Tablets (e.g. Ortho Cyclen®) – Taken once daily.
Transdermal Patch (e.g. Ortho Evra®) – Applied once weekly.
Intravaginal Ring (e.g. NuvaRing®) – Inserted and left in place for three weeks.

**HECKMAN'S
NURSING PHARMACOLOGY SIMPLIFIED**

PROGESTIN-ONLY CONTRACEPTIVES

SELECT EXAMPLES
Ortho Micronor® (norethindrone tablets)
Depo-Provera® (medroxyprogesterone intramuscular injection)
Mirena (levonorgestrel intrauterine device)

Mechanism: Progestin-only contraceptives thicken cervical mucus, suppress ovulation (sometimes), and alter the endometrium to create conditions unfavorable to sperm penetration, fertilization, and implantation.

Common Uses: Prevention of pregnancy

OVULATION *and* FAILURE RATE
Unlike combination products, progestin-only contraceptives do not reliably inhibit ovulation. For example, ovulation occurs in about half of patients who take Ortho Micronor®. This may explain the difference in failure rate. Combination oral hormone contraceptives have a failure rate of about 0.1% per year (with perfect use), while progestin-only oral contraceptives have a failure rate of about 0.5% per year (with perfect use).

NO ESTROGEN-RELATED SIDE EFFECTS
✓ No thromboembolic events   ✓ Lower cancer risk
✓ Less nausea & breast tenderness

THE MOST COMMON SIDE EFFECT
#1 Irregular menstrual bleeding
This explains why progestin-only contraceptives are less commonly prescribed.
Patients are more likely to tolerate nausea and breast tenderness over irregular menstrual bleeding.

DRUG CLASS *of* CHOICE *for* CONTRACEPTION WHILE BREASTFEEDING
NOTE: Estrogen reduces breast milk production in women who are breastfeeding.

SMOKERS OVER 35 YEARS OLD
Because estrogen increases the risk of blood clots, progestin-only contraceptives are safer than combination products for patients who smoke cigarettes and patients who are over the age of 35 years old.

PROGESTINS MAY WORSEN ACNE
Unlike combination hormone contraceptives, which can be used to treat acne, some progestins possess a high level of androgenic activity (e.g. norgestrel, levonorgestrel) that can actually worsen acne.

PREGNANCY CATEGORY X

A VARIETY OF CONVENIENT DOSAGE FORMS
Intramuscular injection (e.g. Depo-Provera®) – Administered once every 90 days.
Subdermal implant (e.g. Nexplanon®) – Inserted and left in place for up to three years.
Intrauterine device (e.g. Mirena®) – Inserted and left in place for up to five years.

AROMATASE INHIBITORS

COMMON EXAMPLES
Arimidex® (anastrozole)   Aromasin® (exemestane)   Femara® (letrozole)

Mechanism: Aromatase inhibitors block the enzyme aromatase which normally converts androgens to estrogen, ultimately reducing estrogen concentrations in the bloodstream.

Common Uses: Hormone receptor-positive breast cancer (postmenopausal women only)

↓ ESTROGEN BY 75–95%
for POSTMENOPAUSAL WOMEN

In premenopausal women, most estrogen is produced by the ovaries. In postmenopausal women, who produce relatively little estrogen, most of the estrogen comes from the activity of aromatase, which converts adrenal androgens to estrogen. Generally, aromatase inhibitors offer no benefit to premenopausal women because aromatase is a relatively minor source of estrogen in this population.

CHOLESTEROL and BONE DENSITY

Reducing the production of estrogen can have many consequences. Just as women may experience an increase in cholesterol and a decrease in bone mineral density with menopause, they may also experience these as a consequence of reducing estrogen production with an aromatase inhibitor.

ELEVATED CHOLESTEROL
Cholesterol monitoring (e.g. fasting lipid panel) may be necessary.

DECREASED BONE DENSITY
Monitoring of bone mineral density may be necessary.

HOT FLASHES
THE #1 SIDE EFFECT of AROMATASE INHIBITORS

During perimenopause and menopause, estrogen production declines and many women experience hot flashes. Similarly, estrogen production declines when the enzyme aromatase is inhibited. Unsurprisingly, hot flashes are the most common side effect of this drug class.

PREGNANCY CATEGORY X
Aromatase inhibitors can cause spontaneous abortion and congenital birth defects, and they should never be used by women who are pregnant.

**HECKMAN'S
NURSING PHARMACOLOGY SIMPLIFIED**

GLUCOCORTICOIDS

COMMON EXAMPLES
Cortef® (hydrocortisone)   Sterapred® (prednisone)   Orapred® (prednisolone)
Medrol® (methylprednisolone)   Decadron® (dexamethasone)

Mechanism: Glucocorticoids bind to glucocorticoid receptors, reducing production of inflammatory mediators and suppressing immune system activity.

Common Uses: Inflammation, allergic reactions, autoimmune disorders, adrenal insufficiency

COMMON SIDE EFFECTS
Emotional lability, insomnia, gastrointestinal (GI) irritation/ulcer, fluid retention, hypertension, hyperglycemia, weight gain, increased intraocular pressure/glaucoma, cataracts, osteoporosis, and thinning of the skin.
NOTE: The likelihood and severity of side effects increase with dose and duration of treatment.

HOW TO REDUCE GI IRRITATION *and* PEPTIC ULCER RISK
Administer each dose with food or milk ± antacids between meals

CORTICOSTEROID WITHDRAWAL
The body produces about 20 mg of hydrocortisone ("cortisol") daily at baseline. Use of medicinal glucocorticoids eventually suppresses physiological production of hydrocortisone. Once this occurs, abrupt discontinuation of the glucocorticoid can lead to corticosteroid withdrawal symptoms (e.g. fever, muscle aches, joint pain, malaise). To reduce the likelihood of withdrawal symptoms, the dose should be tapered (i.e. gradually decreased) over several days.

STRATEGIES *for* AVOIDING WITHDRAWAL

ADMINISTER DAILY DOSES BEFORE 9 AM
During therapy, we can reduce the development of dependence on glucocorticoids by giving once daily doses in the morning before 9 AM. For patients receiving multiple daily doses, the doses should be evenly spaced throughout the day.

TAPER THE DOSE WHEN DISCONTINUING
The likelihood of corticosteroid withdrawal symptoms can be minimized by reducing the glucocorticoid dose gradually over several days, provides time for the body to adjust and start producing normal levels of hydrocortisone again.

POTENTIAL CONSEQUENCES *of* IMMUNOSUPPRESSION

| IMPAIRED WOUND HEALING | INCREASED SUSCEPTIBILITY TO INFECTION | MASKING OF SIGNS OF INFECTION |

NOTE: Do not administer live vaccines to patients receiving immunosuppressive doses of corticosteroids.

CONSIDERATIONS *for* TOPICAL STEROIDS

THINNING OF THE SKIN
The most common side effect associated with topical steroids, particularly with chronic use, is thinning of the skin at the application site.

SYSTEMIC ABSORPTION
To reduce systemic absorption, the application site should not be covered (e.g. with bandages or wraps) unless physician instructs otherwise.

HECKMAN'S
NURSING PHARMACOLOGY SIMPLIFIED

MINERALOCORTICOIDS

THE ONLY COMMERCIALLY AVAILABLE OPTION
Florinef® (fludrocortisone)

Mechanism: Mineralocorticoids exert their effect on the distal convoluted tubule of the kidney, increasing sodium and water reabsorption while simultaneously increasing the excretion of potassium.

Common Uses: Adrenal insufficiency (e.g. Addison's disease)

FLUDROCORTISONE: THE OTHER CORTICOSTEROID
Corticosteroids can be divided into two categories; glucocorticoids, which are known primarily for their anti-inflammatory effects, and mineralocorticoids, which are known for causing sodium and fluid retention. The primary mineralocorticoid produced by the body is aldosterone. Fludrocortisone is the only pharmaceutical mineralocorticoid currently available in the United States.

THE OPPOSITE *of* A POTASSIUM-SPARING DIURETIC
Fludrocortisone mimics aldosterone, the primary mineralocorticoid produced by the human body. Contrast this with potassium-sparing diuretics (e.g. spironolactone), a class of antihypertensive drugs that work by antagonizing aldosterone.

MINERALOCORTICOIDS	POTASSIUM-SPARING DIURETICS
↑ Sodium & Fluid Retention	↓ Sodium & Fluid Retention
↓ Potassium Levels	↑ Potassium Levels

MOST COMMON SIDE EFFECTS
The most common side effects of mineralocorticoids are direct consequences of sodium and fluid retention:
✓ Hypertension   ✓ Edema   ✓ Congestive Heart Failure   ✓ Cardiac Enlargement   ✓ Hypokalemia

NOTE: With high doses or prolonged use, mineralocorticoids produce glucocorticoid-like side effects.

CORTICOSTEROIDS
The image below represents the spectrum of effects associated with corticosteroids. As previously mentioned, glucocorticoids are known for their anti-inflammatory effects and mineralocorticoids are known for inducing sodium and fluid retention.

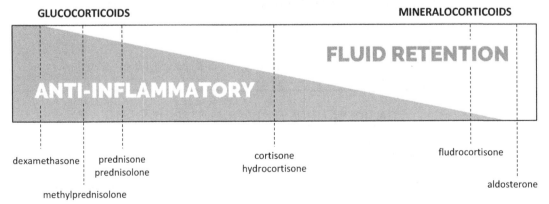

HECKMAN'S
NURSING PHARMACOLOGY SIMPLIFIED

LOOP DIURETICS

COMMON EXAMPLES
Bumex® (bumetanide)   Edecrin® (ethacrynic acid)
Demadex® (torsemide)   Lasix® (furosemide)

Mechanism: Loop diuretics block the reabsorption of sodium ions in the Loop of Henle, the proximal convoluted tubule, and the distal convoluted tubule. The elevated concentration of sodium in the filtrate osmotically draws additional water into the urine, thereby reducing blood volume and blood pressure.

Common Uses: Edema, hypertension

THE GREATEST DIURETIC EFFECT
Of the three major classes of diuretics (loop, thiazide, and potassium-sparing diuretics), loop diuretics exert the greatest diuretic effect.

SIX-HOUR DURATION *of* ACTION
Orally administered Lasix® "**la**sts **six** hours." Coincidentally, all orally administered loop diuretics last for about six hours.

EXCESSIVE URINATION
Excessive urination is the most common side effect of loop diuretics. To prevent nocturia, patients should take loop diuretics early in the day. Patients on a twice-daily dosing regimen should take the first dose in the morning and the second dose in the early afternoon (e.g. 8 AM and 2 PM).

HYPOKALEMIA
While promoting renal excretion of sodium, the use of loop diuretics commonly results in the loss other electrolytes, especially potassium.

HYPERGLYCEMIA
Loop diuretics may cause minor increases in blood glucose levels, which may require insulin adjustment for patients with diabetes.

BLACK BOX WARNING
Excessive doses of loop diuretics can cause severe electrolyte and water depletion.

OTOTOXICITY
High doses of loop diuretics, particularly in patients with severe renal impairment, have been associated with hearing loss, tinnitus, and vertigo. The risk of these ototoxic effects is greater in patients who are receiving other ototoxic medications, such as aminoglycosides.

MONITORING PARAMETERS
✓Renal function   ✓Electrolytes   ✓Blood glucose

NOTE: Body weight monitoring may be necessary for patients with congestive heart failure, and blood pressure should be monitored when used for hypertension.

HECKMAN'S
NURSING PHARMACOLOGY SIMPLIFIED

THIAZIDE DIURETICS

THE MOST COMMON EXAMPLE
Microzide® (hydrochlorothiazide)

Mechanism: Thiazide diuretics block the reabsorption of sodium ions in the distal convoluted tubule. The elevated concentration of sodium in the filtrate osmotically draws additional water into the urine, thereby reducing blood volume and blood pressure.

Common Uses: Hypertension, edema

MAJOR SIMILARITIES TO LOOP DIURETICS

ADMINISTER EARLY IN THE DAY
As with loop diuretics, thiazide diuretics should be administered early in the day to prevent nocturia.

HYPOKALEMIA
As with loop diuretics, the use of thiazide diuretics commonly results in the loss other electrolytes, especially potassium.

HYPERGLYCEMIA
Thiazide diuretics can produce minor elevations in blood glucose, which may require insulin adjustment for patients with diabetes.

NOTE: Loop and thiazide diuretics can be categorized more broadly as "potassium-depleting diuretics."

MONITORING PARAMETERS
✓ Renal function ✓ Electrolytes ✓ Blood glucose

NOTE: Blood pressure should also be monitored periodically when used for the treatment of hypertension.

MAJOR DIFFERENCES *from* LOOP DIURETICS

DURATION *of* ACTION
Thiazide diuretics have a longer duration of action than loop diuretics, making them more suitable for treatment of chronic conditions like hypertension.

DIURETIC EFFECT
Thiazide diuretics are less effective than loop diuretics, but more effective than potassium-sparing diuretics.

THERAPEUTIC USE
Thiazide diuretics are typically used to treat hypertension; whereas, loop diuretics are typically used to treat edema.

SITE *of* ACTION
Thiazide diuretics block sodium reabsorption in one part of the nephron—the distal convoluted tubule; meanwhile, loop diuretics block sodium reabsorption in the Loop of Henle, the proximal convoluted tubule, and the distal convoluted tubule. This explains why thiazide diuretics produce a milder effect, and why thiazide diuretics don't carry the same black box warning as loop diuretics.

HECKMAN'S
NURSING PHARMACOLOGY SIMPLIFIED

POTASSIUM-SPARING DIURETICS

THE MOST COMMON EXAMPLE
Aldactone® (spironolactone)

Mechanism: Spironolactone antagonizes aldosterone receptors in the distal convoluted tubule, ultimately increasing renal excretion of sodium and water while retaining potassium.

Common Uses: Hypertension, edema, primary hyperaldosteronism

DIURETIC EFFECT
Of the three major classes of diuretics (loop, thiazide, and potassium-sparing diuretics), potassium-sparing diuretics exert the **weakest** diuretic effect.

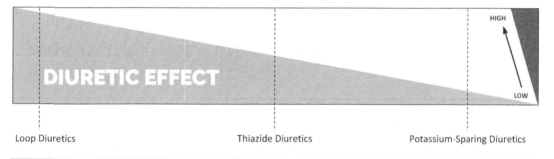

Loop Diuretics Thiazide Diuretics Potassium-Sparing Diuretics

---

SERUM POTASSIUM LEVELS
Potassium depletion is the biggest potential problem associated with the use of loop and thiazide diuretics. On the flip side, potassium-sparing diuretics can cause hyperkalemia, particularly when used with substances that increase serum potassium levels, such as potassium supplements, angiotensin-converting enzyme inhibitors, and angiotensin II receptor blockers.

AVOID SALT SUBSTITUTES
Salt substitutes typically contain potassium, increasing the risk of hyperkalemia.

MONITOR ELECTROLYTES
Never administer potassium-sparing diuretics to a patient with hyperkalemia.

ADD-ON THERAPY TO A POTASSIUM DEPLETING DIURETIC
When response to a potassium-depleting diuretic (e.g. hydrochlorothiazide) is inadequate, a potassium-sparing diuretic can be added for the dual benefit of boosting diuresis and counteracting potassium depletion.

ANTI-ANDROGENIC PROPERTIES

RISK OF GYNECOMASTIA
Male breast development (gynecomastia) is the most common side effect of spironolactone affecting about 1 in 11 men.

AVOID DURING PREGNANCY
Spironolactone opposes the activity of testosterone, potentially interfering with prenatal development of male sex characteristics.

MONITOR RENAL FUNCTION
Diuretics are eliminated largely by the kidneys. Doses may need to be reduced in cases of renal impairment.

**HECKMAN'S
NURSING PHARMACOLOGY SIMPLIFIED**

ACE INHIBITORS and ARBs

ANGIOTENSIN CONVERTING ENZYME INHIBITORS (ACE INHIBITORS)
Prinivil®, Zestril® (lisinopril), Vasotec® (enalapril)
Altace® (ramipril), Lotensin® (benazepril)

Drug Name Stem: –pril

ANGIOTENSIN II RECEPTOR BLOCKERS (ARBs)
Cozaar® (losartan), Diovan® (valsartan)
Benicar® (olmesartan), Avapro® (irbesartan)

Drug Name Stem: –sartan

THE DRUG TARGET: ANGIOTENSIN II
Angiotensin II is a hormone that raises blood pressure mainly by:
1) Binding to and activating receptors in blood vessels, causing them to constrict.
2) Binding to and activating receptors on the adrenal glands, causing them to secrete aldosterone.

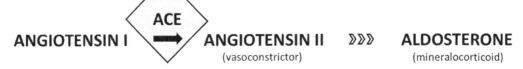

ANGIOTENSIN I →(ACE)→ ANGIOTENSIN II (vasoconstrictor) »»» ALDOSTERONE (mineralocorticoid)

ACE INHIBITORS
ACE inhibitors block ACE, the enzyme that converts the relatively inactive angiotensin I to the highly active angiotensin II.

ARBs
ARBs interfere with the binding of angiotensin II to receptors in key locations such as the blood vessels and adrenal glands.

ACE inhibitors and ARBs ultimately produce the same blood pressure-lowering effects.
EFFECT #1: Reduced angiotensin II-mediated vasoconstriction ⇨ relaxation of blood vessels
EFFECT #2: Reduced angiotensin II-mediated aldosterone secretion ⇨ reduced sodium and fluid retention

---

MAKING SENSE OF THE COMMON SIDE EFFECTS
✓Dizziness ✓Headache ✓Hypotension ✓Hyperkalemia ✓Dry Cough*

Hypotension, dizziness, and headache are typical consequences of vasodilation. Elevated potassium levels are a direct consequence of reduced aldosterone secretion (*see page 84 for more on aldosterone*).

*Dry cough is a side effect unique to ACE inhibitors. ACE plays a key role in the degradation of bradykinins (a class of inflammatory mediators). When ACE is inhibited, the resultant accumulation of bradykinins can trigger a persistent dry cough. Since ARBs do not inhibit ACE, they do not interfere with the degradation of bradykinins. When a patient develops a dry cough while taking an ACE inhibitor, it is common for the practitioner to replace the ACE inhibitor with an ARB.

DO NOT ADMINISTER DURING PREGNANCY
Due to the risk of fetal injury and death, ACE inhibitors and ARBs should not be used during pregnancy except in very rare situations where the use of an ACE inhibitor or ARB is necessary to save the life of the mother.

ADMINISTER WITH *or* WITHOUT FOOD
ACE inhibitors and ARBs can be administered with or without food.

HECKMAN'S
NURSING PHARMACOLOGY SIMPLIFIED

BETA-BLOCKERS

COMMON EXAMPLES
Lopressor® (metoprolol tartrate)   Toprol® XL (metoprolol succinate)   Tenormin® (atenolol)
Coreg® (carvedilol)   Inderal® (propranolol)

Drug Name Stem: –lol

Mechanism: Beta-blockers antagonize beta-adrenergic receptors in cardiac muscle tissue, which reduces heart rate, cardiac contractility, and blood pressure.

Common Uses: Hypertension, atrial fibrillation, reduction of cardiovascular mortality after a heart attack, migraine prophylaxis, essential tremor

ADMINISTER WITH FOOD
Generally, administering a beta-blocker with food will result in slower absorption and may reduce the incidence of side effects such as postural hypotension.

PATIENTS SHOULD NOT DISCONTINUE ABRUPTLY
Abrupt discontinuation of a beta-blocker can lead to severe exacerbations of angina, ventricular arrhythmias, and myocardial infarctions. The dose should be reduced slowly over a period of 1–2 weeks. Advise patients to minimize physical activity during this period and only discontinue a beta-blocker with the advice of a physician.

COMMON BETA-BLOCKER SIDE EFFECTS
✓Fatigue   ✓Dizziness   ✓Bradycardia*   ✓Hypotension**   ✓Shortness of Breath

*MONITOR HEART RATE (HR)
Notify physician if HR < 50 beats/minute

**MONITOR BLOOD PRESSURE (BP)
Notify physician if systolic BP < 100 mmHg

WARNING *for* PATIENTS WITH DIABETES
Beta-blockers can mask several signs of hypoglycemia, including tachycardia and tremors.
Sweating is one of the few signs of hypoglycemia that is not masked by a beta-blocker.

NONSELECTIVE BETA-BLOCKERS
Inderal® (propranolol), Normodyne® (labetalol), Coreg® (carvedilol), Betapace® (sotalol)

CARDIOSELECTIVE BETA-BLOCKERS
Lopressor® (metoprolol), Tenormin (atenolol), Zebeta® (bisoprolol), Bystolic® (nebivolol)

The cardioselective beta-blockers preferentially antagonize $beta_1$ receptors (located in the heart); whereas, nonselective beta-blockers indiscriminately antagonize $beta_1$ and $beta_2$ receptors (located in the lungs). Patients with asthma or chronic obstructive pulmonary disease (COPD) typically rely on inhaled **$beta_2$ agonists** (e.g. albuterol) to dilate the airways for improved breathing. For $beta_2$ agonists to dilate the airways, they must first bind to $beta_2$ receptors; however, if $beta_2$ receptors are blocked, the requisite binding cannot take place. For this reason, cardioselective beta-blockers are generally preferred for patients with asthma or COPD.

NOTE: All beta-blockers are class II antiarrhythmics.

HECKMAN'S
NURSING PHARMACOLOGY SIMPLIFIED

ALPHA-BLOCKERS

COMMON EXAMPLES
Cardura® (doxazosin)   Hytrin® (terazosin)   Minipress® (prazosin)
Flomax® (tamsulosin)   Rapaflo® (silodosin)

Drug Name Stem: –osin

Mechanism: Alpha-blockers antagonize alpha$_1$ adrenergic receptors, opposing the activity of adrenergic hormones (e.g. adrenaline).

Common Uses: Benign prostatic hyperplasia (BPH), hypertension

ALPHA$_1$ RECEPTOR SUBTYPES: ALPHA$_{1A}$ & ALPHA$_{1B}$
Among the alpha$_1$ receptor subtypes, there are two that can be targeted for medical purposes. The first is alpha$_{1A}$, which mediates smooth muscle contraction in the prostate and bladder neck. The second is alpha$_{1B}$, which mediates smooth muscle contraction in the blood vessels.

NON-SUBTYPE-SELECTIVE ALPHA$_1$ ANTAGONISTS
Doxazosin, terazosin, and prazosin antagonize both alpha$_{1A}$ and alpha$_{1B}$ receptors in the prostate gland and vascular smooth muscle, respectively. They can be used to treat BPH and hypertension; however, they are more likely to cause cardiovascular side effects (e.g. postural hypotension, edema, and dizziness).

ALPHA$_{1A}$ SUBTYPE-SELECTIVE ANTAGONISTS
Tamsulosin and silodosin selectively antagonize the alpha$_{1A}$ receptor subtype, which is predominantly located in the prostate gland. Consequently, they can be used to treat BPH, but not hypertension. They are more likely to cause prostate-related side effects (e.g. retrograde ejaculation), but less likely to cause cardiovascular side effects.

THE FIRST-DOSE EFFECT
The first dose of an alpha-blocker may cause excessive hypotension and fainting. Although this "first-dose effect" can occur with any alpha-blocker, it is more likely to occur with a non-subtype-selective agent (doxazosin, terazosin, or prazosin). To avoid the first-dose effect, doxazosin, terazosin, and prazosin are initiated at a low bedtime dose; then the dose is increased gradually over the course of several days or weeks. Administering the first dose when the patient is in bed eliminates the risk of injury from falling.

COMMON OFF-LABEL USES

Minipress® (prazosin)
Treatment of PTSD-associated nightmares.

Flomax® (tamsulosin)
Promotes the passage of ureteral stones.

FIRST-LINE TREATMENT *for* BPH
✓ Flomax® (tamsulosin)
The most commonly used medication for the treatment of BPH.
Take 30 minutes following the same meal each day.

HECKMAN'S
NURSING PHARMACOLOGY SIMPLIFIED

ALPHA$_2$ AGONISTS

COMMON EXAMPLES
Catapres® (clonidine)   Aldomet® (methyldopa)   Zanaflex® (tizanidine)

Mechanism: Alpha$_2$ agonists activate alpha$_2$ receptors in the central nervous system, reducing sympathetic nervous system (adrenergic) output.

Common Uses: Hypertension (clonidine and methyldopa), muscle spasms (tizanidine), attention deficit/hyperactivity disorder (clonidine)

COMMON SIDE EFFECTS
✓ Dry Mouth   ✓ Drowsiness/sedation

Sedation is a logical consequence of reducing sympathetic nervous system activity. Advise patients to avoid driving and operating machinery until the effects are known. Sedation is most likely to occur early in treatment/with dose increases and may diminish as tolerance develops.

OTHER POTENTIAL SIDE EFFECTS
✓ Bradycardia   ✓ Hypotension

NOTE: Monitor heart rate and blood pressure periodically.

PATIENTS SHOULD NOT DISCONTINUE ABRUPTLY
DUE TO RISK *of* REBOUND HYPERTENSION *and* WITHDRAWAL SYMPTOMS

Rebound hypertension and withdrawal symptoms including tachycardia, tremor, nervousness, agitation, and sweating can occur with abrupt discontinuation of an alpha$_2$ agonist, particularly when used for ≥ 2 months. To discontinue, follow the advice of a physician and reduce the dose gradually over several days.

ALDOMET® (METHYLDOPA)
THE DRUG *of* CHOICE *for* HYPERTENSION DURING PREGNANCY

Methyldopa is relatively safe and effective during pregnancy. Keep in-mind that most pregnant women take prenatal vitamins that contain iron, and iron can reduce the absorption and effect of methyldopa. Separate administration of prenatal vitamins (or iron supplements) from methyldopa by at least two hours.

INSTRUCT PATIENTS TO
AVOID ALCOHOLIC BEVERAGES

The sedative effects of alpha$_2$ agonists are enhanced by alcohol and other sedating drugs (e.g. opioids, benzodiazepines, barbiturates).

HECKMAN'S
NURSING PHARMACOLOGY SIMPLIFIED

CALCIUM CHANNEL BLOCKERS

COMMON EXAMPLES
Norvasc® (amlodipine)   Procardia®, Adalat CC® (nifedipine)   Cardene® (nicardipine)
Cardizem®, Cartia XT®, Tiazac® (diltiazem)   Calan®, Isoptin®, Verelan® (verapamil)

Drug Name Stem: –dipine*

Mechanism: Calcium channel blockers inhibit the influx of calcium ions into cardiac and vascular smooth muscle tissue. This results in dilated blood vessels, reduced heart rate, and reduced cardiac contractility.

Common Uses: Hypertension, angina, cardiac arrhythmias (diltiazem and verapamil)

THE #1 SIDE EFFECT: HEADACHE
This and many other side effects of calcium channel blockers can be attributed to vasodilation. Dilated blood vessels in the head can press on pain receptors (nociceptors), causing a headache. Other common side effects that can be a consequence of vasodilation include peripheral edema, hypotension, dizziness, and flushing.

INSTRUCT PATIENTS TO
AVOID GRAPEFRUIT JUICE
Grapefruit juice contains compounds that inhibit a key metabolic enzyme involved in the elimination of many calcium channel blockers. Consequently, it is prudent to advise patients not to consume grapefruit or grapefruit juice while taking a calcium channel blocker.

DILTIAZEM *and* VERAPAMIL
Diltiazem and verapamil are "Non-Dihydropyridine Calcium Channel Blockers." Compared to other drugs in this class, these two have a more pronounced effect on cardiac tissue, making them more useful for situations that require reduction in heart rate and cardiac contractility. All other calcium channel blockers (e.g. amlodipine, nifedipine, nicardipine) are "Dihydropyridine Calcium Channel Blockers." These drugs exert their effect predominantly on vascular smooth muscle cells, making them more useful in situations where vasodilation is the primary goal.

CLASS IV ANTIARRHYTHMICS
Due to their pronounced effect on heart rate and cardiac contractility, diltiazem and verapamil are used for treating cardiac arrhythmias.

BLOOD PRESSURE *and* HEART RATE
Diltiazem and verapamil are contraindicated when systolic blood pressure is < 90 mmHg. Also, monitor for bradycardia (heart rate < 50 bpm).

*****NOTE:** The only drugs in this class that do not end in "–dipine" are diltiazem and verapamil, which are the non-dihydropyridine calcium channel blockers. All others that end in "–dipine" are dihydropyridine calcium channel blockers. The drug name stem "–dipine" is essentially an abbreviation for "dihydropyridine."

ORGANIC NITRATES

COMMON EXAMPLES
Nitrostat® (nitroglycerin sublingual tablets)   Nitrolingual® (nitroglycerin lingual spray)
Nitro-Bid® (nitroglycerin ointment)   Nitro-Dur® (nitroglycerin transdermal patch)
Imdur® (isosorbide mononitrate)   Isordil® (isosorbide dinitrate)

Mechanism: Organic nitrates dilate veins and arteries (including coronary arteries) by relaxing vascular smooth muscle tissue. This reduces myocardial oxygen demand and increases blood flow to the heart.

Common Uses: Angina treatment and prevention

THE #1 SIDE EFFECT: HEADACHE
As with other drugs that dilate blood vessels, the most common side effect is headache. This occurs when dilated blood vessels press on nociceptors in the head. Reflex tachycardia can also occur as the heart beats faster to compensate for the reduced blood pressure. Other common side effects linked to low blood pressure and vasodilation include dizziness and flushing.

ACUTE ANGINA EPISODES
Nitroglycerin is effective for treating acute episodes of angina when given as an intravenous infusion, sublingual tablet (1–3-minute onset of action), or lingual spray. Other routes of administration, like the ointment or patch, do not enter the blood stream fast enough to treat acute episodes.

NITROSTAT®
Sublingual tablets are the most commonly used form of nitroglycerin. Remind patients to let the medication sit under the tongue. When swallowed, nitroglycerin is quickly deactivated by the liver. Store the tablets at room temperature, tightly sealed in the original glass bottle. Advise patients against storing the medication in warm places, like in their pants pocket. Nitroglycerin is a volatile substance that is prone to evaporate.

TAKE SITTING DOWN
Nitroglycerin can cause hypotension and syncope. To prevent falls, instruct the patient to sit down prior to administering nitroglycerin.

PREVENTION of ANGINA
Organic nitrates used for prevention of angina include Nitro-Bid® (nitroglycerin ointment), Nitro-Dur® (nitroglycerin transdermal patch), Imdur® (isosorbide mononitrate), and Isordil® (isosorbide dinitrate). These formulations have a slower onset of action, but a longer duration of action.

TOLERANCE
Tolerance to organic nitrates develops quickly. After about 12–14 hours of exposure, the anti-anginal effect begins to disappear.

NITRATE-FREE PERIOD
To avoid tolerance, any daily dosing regimen for an organic nitrate should include a daily 10–12-hour nitrate-free period. Fortunately, the products in this category are designed to facilitate this. For example, the isosorbide extended-release formulations are designed to be given once daily and exert an effect for 12 hours, and Nitro-Dur® is designed for a 12–14-hour patch-on period followed by a 10–12-hour patch-off period.

DRUG INTERACTION WITH PDE-5 INHIBITORS
Organic nitrates should never be taken with PDE-5 inhibitors like Viagra® (sildenafil), Cialis® (tadalafil), or Levitra® (vardenafil). This combination can cause fatal hypotension or heart attack.

PDE-5 INHIBITORS

COMMON EXAMPLES
Viagra® (sildenafil)   Cialis® (tadalafil)   Levitra® (vardenafil)

Drug Name Stem: –afil

Mechanism: PDE-5 inhibitors block the enzyme phosphodiesterase-5 (PDE-5), enhancing the effect of nitric oxide predominantly in the corpus cavernosum.

Common Uses: Erectile dysfunction (ED)

SPECIAL ADMINISTRATION INSTRUCTIONS
Take as needed approximately one hour (60 minutes) prior to sexual activity.
NOTE: Maximum one dose per day.

HEADACHE *and* FLUSHING
THE MOST COMMON SIDE EFFECTS
Headache and flushing are the two most common side effects, which is logical given that PDE-5 inhibitors cause vasodilation. Dilated cranial blood vessels can press on nearby nociceptors and cause a headache. As for flushing, this is a consequence of blood rushing to areas where blood vessels are dilated—in this case, dilation of blood vessels near the surface of the skin.

PDE-5 INHIBITORS + NITRATES
A POTENTIALLY DEADLY DRUG COMBINATION
PDE-5 inhibitors (e.g. sildenafil, tadalafil, vardenafil) and nitrates (e.g. nitroglycerin, isosorbide mononitrate, isosorbide dinitrate) cause vasodilation. For this reason, PDE-5 inhibitors and nitrates should never be used at the same time, as this could result in life-threatening hypotension.

PRIAPISM RISK
EMERGENCY MEDICAL ATTENTION REQUIRED *for* PROLONGED ERECTIONS
Though rare, PDE-5 inhibitors carry the risk of priapism—a painful erection that lasts for more than four hours. Without treatment, priapism can cause permanent tissue damage and impotence. Advise patients to seek emergency medical attention if they have an erection that lasts more than four hours.

BPH
BENIGN PROSTATIC HYPERPLASIA
Cialis® (tadalafil) is also FDA-approved for the treatment of erectile dysfunction and BPH.

PAH
PULMONARY ARTERIAL HYPERTENSION
Revatio® (sildenafil) is FDA-approved for the treatment of pulmonary arterial hypertension.

ANTIARRHYTHMICS

COMMON EXAMPLES
Xylocaine® (lidocaine)   Cordarone® (amiodarone)   Betapace® (sotalol)

Mechanism: Antiarrhythmics alter conduction of cardiac nerve impulses.

Common Uses: Cardiac arrhythmias

ELECTROLYTE ABNORMALITIES
MUST BE CORRECTED TO MINIMIZE THE PROBABILITY of EXACERBATING AN ARRHYTHMIA
All antiarrhythmics can cause or exacerbate cardiac arrhythmias, potentially leading to deadly ventricular arrhythmia and cardiac arrest. Electrolyte levels should be checked, and potassium or magnesium deficiencies should be corrected prior to initiating an antiarrhythmic drug.

ELECTROCARDIOGRAM MONITORING
REQUIRED for MANY of the COMMON ANTIARRHYTHMICS
As mentioned previously, all antiarrhythmics can cause or exacerbate cardiac arrhythmias. Consequently, a certain amount of electrocardiogram monitoring is typically required with these drugs.

LIDOCAINE	AMIODARONE	SOTALOL
Continuous electrocardiogram (ECG) monitoring is required during administration.	Hospitalization and ECG monitoring are required for the loading dose.	Three days of hospitalization and ECG monitoring are required to start or re-start.

POTENTIALLY SEVERE TOXICITIES

LIDOCAINE
Lidocaine can be fatally toxic at plasma concentrations above 6 mcg/mL. It should only be used for the acute management of ventricular arrhythmias. Lidocaine toxicity is characterized by sedation and/or muscle twitching and can progress to seizures and respiratory depression/arrest. Be prepared with equipment to establish an artificial airway and ventilation.

AMIODARONE
Amiodarone has many potentially toxic effects and should be reserved only for the treatment of life-threatening ventricular arrhythmias. Potential toxicities affect the lungs, liver, thyroid gland, eyes, and nerve cells. Patients taking amiodarone must receive routine chest x-rays, pulmonary function tests, liver function tests, thyroid function tests, eye exams, and other tests when clinically indicated.

PATIENTS SHOULD NOT DISCONTINUE SOTALOL ABRUPTLY
Sotalol has two antiarrhythmic mechanisms of action. It works by blocking beta receptors and by blocking potassium channels. Since sotalol has beta-blocker properties, patients should be warned that abrupt discontinuation could lead to a heart attack.

NOTE: Beta-blockers (see page 89) and calcium channel blockers (see page 92) are also antiarrhythmics.

**HECKMAN'S
NURSING PHARMACOLOGY SIMPLIFIED**

DIGITALIS GLYCOSIDES

THE MOST COMMON EXAMPLE
Lanoxin® (digoxin)

Mechanism: Digoxin inhibits sodium/potassium ATPase (Na^+/K^+ ATPase), ultimately increasing the concentration of intracellular calcium in cardiac muscle cells.

Common Uses: Congestive heart failure (CHF), atrial fibrillation (AFib)

DIGOXIN THERAPEUTIC APPLICATIONS

Digoxin serum concentrations from 0.5–2.0 ng/mL are therapeutic and levels above 2.0 ng/mL are usually toxic. At lower concentrations, digoxin is effective for treating CHF. Higher concentrations are effective for treating AFib. Not every patient will experience therapeutic or toxic effects at the thresholds outlined below, so the dose should be adjusted based on a combination of signs of improvement, signs of toxicity, and digoxin serum concentrations.

THERAPEUTIC CONCENTRATION *for* CHF	THERAPEUTIC CONCENTRATION *for* AFib
0.5–0.9 ng/mL	0.8–2.0 ng/mL

TOXIC CONCENTRATION
> 2.0 ng/mL

DIGOXIN TOXICITY

Digoxin toxicity is characterized by nausea/vomiting, visual disturbances (e.g. green-yellow color disturbances, halo effect), and cardiac arrhythmias. This usually occurs when digoxin serum concentrations exceed 2.0 ng/mL.

MONITOR ELECTROLYTES
LOW K^+, LOW Mg^{2+}, or HIGH Ca^{2+} INCREASE THE RISK *of* TOXICITY

Electrolyte levels should be checked at baseline and then periodically throughout treatment. Hypokalemia, hypomagnesemia, and hypercalcemia can all increase the risk of digoxin toxicity. Deficiencies in potassium or magnesium should be corrected.

HR | # BP

Patients should be instructed to monitor and maintain a daily record of their heart rate (HR). | Patients should be instructed to monitor and maintain a daily record of their blood pressure (BP).

THE ANTIDOTE *for* DIGOXIN

Digibind® and DigiFab® (digoxin immune fab), antibody fragments that bind and remove digoxin from the bloodstream.

POTASSIUM CHLORIDE

COMMON EXAMPLES
Klor-Con®, K-Dur® (potassium chloride) Potassium chloride injection

Mechanism: Potassium is an electrolyte with a key role in several physiological functions, including nerve impulse transmission and cardiac, skeletal, and smooth muscle contraction.

Common Uses: Hypokalemia treatment and prevention

NOTE: The normal serum concentration of potassium is 3.5–5.0 mEq/L.

ORAL (PO) DOSAGE FORMS

GASTROINTESTINAL (GI) IRRITATION
Orally administered potassium chloride can be irritating to the GI tract. Consequently, common side effects include nausea/vomiting, abdominal pain, flatulence, diarrhea, and GI bleeding.

SOLID ORAL DOSAGE FORMS
Oral potassium tablets and capsules should be taken with a meal and a full glass of water to reduce GI irritation. Also, patients should avoid splitting, crushing, and chewing the tablets and capsules.

LIQUID ORAL DOSAGE FORMS
Oral potassium solutions and powders must be diluted with liquid according to package instructions prior to administration, and the resulting mixture should be consumed slowly over several minutes.

INTRAVENOUS (IV) DOSAGE FORMS

EXTRAVASATION RISK
Just as oral potassium chloride irritates the GI tract, injectable potassium chloride can irritate the vein and surrounding tissue. Administration through a peripheral line is commonly associated with pain and phlebitis, and extravasation can result in ulceration and necrosis. To reduce the incidence of pain, phlebitis, and extravasation, administration through a central venous catheter is generally preferred.

HIGH ALERT MEDICATION
Inappropriate preparation and administration of potassium chloride injection can lead to potentially fatal cardiac arrhythmias and cardiac arrest.

NEVER ADMINISTER CONCENTRATED PRODUCT
Injectable potassium chloride must be diluted prior to administration. Never administer potassium chloride directly from a vial or with a label indicating the product is concentrated. Intravenous administration of undiluted potassium (e.g. as an IV push) can cause cardiac arrest.

NEVER ADMINISTER A RAPID INFUSION
Potassium chloride must be infused slowly, typically at a rate of 10 mEq/hour in adults. In urgent or severe cases, potassium chloride can be infused at a rate of 40 mEq/hour with continuous cardiac monitoring and frequent monitoring of serum potassium levels.

THE ANTIDOTE for POTASSIUM
Kayexalate® (polystyrene sulfonate), a product that sequesters excess potassium in cases of hyperkalemia.

HECKMAN'S
NURSING PHARMACOLOGY SIMPLIFIED

VASOPRESSORS

COMMON EXAMPLES
Neo-Synephrine® (phenylephrine)   Levophed® (norepinephrine)   Adrenalin® (epinephrine)
Intropin® (dopamine)   Dobutrex® (dobutamine)

Mechanism: Vasopressors stimulate adrenergic receptors (e.g. $alpha_1$, $beta_1$, bet_2 receptors), increasing heart rate (chronotropy), the force of myocardial contractions (inotropy) and/or vasoconstriction.

Common Uses: Acute hypotension (e.g. cardiogenic shock, septic shock)

CORRECT VOLUME DEPLETION
Volume depletion should be corrected with fluid and electrolytes and/or blood or plasma transfusions **before** starting any vasopressor; otherwise, severe vasoconstriction and ischemic injury can occur.

ADMINISTER VIA CENTRAL LINE
Extravasation of vasopressors can cause necrosis due to local vasoconstriction. To reduce the likelihood of extravasation, vasopressors are usually administered through a central venous catheter when possible.

CARDIOVASCULAR EFFECTS

	$Alpha_1$ Activity	$Beta_1$ Activity	$Beta_2$ Activity
phenylephrine	✓		
norepinephrine	✓	✓	
epinephrine	✓	✓	✓
dopamine	✓	✓	
dobutamine		✓	✓

$Alpha_1$ receptor activation causes contraction of the smooth muscle in blood vessels (vasoconstriction). $Beta_1$ receptor activation increases heart rate and cardiac contractility (inotropic and chronotropic effects). $Beta_2$ receptor activation dilates coronary arteries and arteries that supply blood to skeletal muscles.

NOTE: Dopamine also stimulates dopamine receptors, which increases blood flow to the kidneys.

SERIOUS POTENTIAL SIDE EFFECTS

✓Tachycardia   ✓Arrhythmias   ✓Hypertension   ✓Ischemic Injury

CARDIAC MONITORING *for* VASOPRESSORS

BP
BLOOD PRESSURE

HR
HEART RATE

ECG
ELECTROCARDIOGRAM

ADJUST THE FLOW RATE (DOSE) BASED ON THE PATIENT'S BLOOD PRESSURE and HEART RATE

HECKMAN'S
NURSING PHARMACOLOGY SIMPLIFIED

VITAMIN K ANTAGONISTS

THE MOST COMMON EXAMPLE
Coumadin®, Jantoven® (warfarin)

Mechanism: Warfarin antagonizes vitamin K, interfering with the activation of vitamin K-dependent clotting factors (factor II, VII, IX, and X).

Common Uses: Blood clot treatment and prevention

BLEEDING
THE #1 SIDE EFFECT *of* WARFARIN
Can range from minor bleeding to life-threatening hemorrhaging!
NOTE: Monitor patients for signs of bleeding such as black, tarry, or bloody stools, excessive bruising, red or dark brown urine.

WARFARIN + NSAIDs
A MAJOR POTENTIAL DRUG INTERACTION
Non-steroidal anti-inflammatory drugs (NSAIDs) irritate the stomach and can cause gastrointestinal bleeding. Patients on warfarin should not take medications that contain aspirin, ibuprofen, or naproxen without consulting a physician.

4.0
THE INR DANGER ZONE
Warfarin is a narrow therapeutic index drug, and routine INR monitoring is required for safe and effective use. With few exceptions, INR levels greater than 4.0 are associated with a high risk of bleeding with no additional therapeutic benefit.

COLOR-CODED TABLETS
Warfarin tablet color is standardized based on strength.
For example, warfarin 5 mg tablets are always orange, regardless of the brand or manufacturer.

X
PREGNANCY CATEGORY X
Due to the risk of teratogenic and toxic effects to the fetus, warfarin should not be used during pregnancy, **except** by women with mechanical heart valves who are at high risk of thromboembolism.

K
THE ANTIDOTE *for* WARFARIN
Warfarin antagonizes vitamin K, interfering with the activation of vitamin K-dependent clotting factors. Not surprisingly, warfarin can be reversed by administering Vitamin K_1 (phytonadione).

ORAL DIRECT THROMBIN INHIBITORS

THE ONLY EXAMPLE
Pradaxa® (dabigatran)

Mechanism: Direct thrombin inhibitors directly inhibits thrombin, which reduces the amount of fibrinogen that is converted to fibrin, ultimately preventing the development of a thrombus.

Common Uses: Deep vein thrombosis, pulmonary embolism, blood clot risk reduction in patients with nonvalvular atrial fibrillation

---

NO ROUTINE BLOOD TESTS
Pradaxa® (dabigatran) does not require routine blood tests.
This gives dabigatran an advantage over warfarin, which requires routine INR monitoring. However, the convenience comes at a cost; dabigatran is considerably more expensive than warfarin.
NOTE: The dose should be lowered for patients with renal impairment. Monitor renal function periodically.

THE #1 SIDE EFFECT: BLEEDING
Dabigatran can cause bleeding events ranging from minor to life-threatening and is contraindicated in patients with active pathological bleeding. Advise patients to report unusual bruising or bleeding to their physician.

STRESS THE IMPORTANCE *of* TAKING EXACTLY AS PRESCRIBED
Compliance is important with all medications; however, the consequence of failing to take an anticoagulant as prescribed could be fatal. An overdose could cause a life-threatening hemorrhage and missed doses could lead to a thromboembolic event.

ADVISE PATIENTS NOT TO CRUSH/BREAK/CHEW PRADAXA®
Instruct patients to swallow Pradaxa® (dabigatran) capsules whole with a full glass of water. If the capsule shell is not intact, about 75% more dabigatran will be absorbed, which may cause excessive anticoagulation and bleeding.

INSTRUCT PATIENTS NOT TO STORE PRADAXA® IN PILL ORGANIZERS
Pradaxa® (dabigatran) is sensitive to moisture, so the capsules must be stored in the original bottle, which contains a desiccant (drying agent) inside the lid. The medication may also be distributed in blister packs. In any case, do not remove a capsule from the original packaging until immediately prior to administration.

PRADAXA® + NSAIDs = ↑ RISK *of* GASTROINTESTINAL (GI) BLEEDING
Non-steroidal anti-inflammatory drugs (NSAIDs) have the potential to cause GI bleeding directly by irritating the GI mucosa and indirectly by reducing prostaglandin-mediated gastric mucus production. Concurrent use of a drug that interferes with coagulation (e.g. dabigatran) increases this risk of bleeding. Unless instructed otherwise, patients on dabigatran should avoid aspirin, ibuprofen, and naproxen.

THE ANTIDOTE *for* DABIGATRAN
Praxbind® (idarucizumab), a monoclonal antibody fragment that binds and effectively deactivates dabigatran.

HECKMAN'S
NURSING PHARMACOLOGY SIMPLIFIED

ORAL FACTOR Xa INHIBITORS

COMMON EXAMPLES
Eliquis® (apixaban)   Savaysa® (edoxaban)   Xarelto® (rivaroxaban)

Drug Name Stem: –xaban

Mechanism: Factor Xa inhibitors selectively inhibit factor Xa, ultimately reducing thrombin formation and thrombus development.

Common Uses: Deep vein thrombosis, pulmonary embolism, blood clot risk reduction in patients with nonvalvular atrial fibrillation

NO ROUTINE BLOOD TESTS
Factor Xa inhibitors do not require routine blood tests.
Like dabigatran, this gives oral factor Xa inhibitors an advantage over warfarin, which requires routine INR monitoring; however, they are considerably more expensive than warfarin.

NOTE: Dose adjustments may be required for patients with renal impairment.

THE #1 SIDE EFFECT: BLEEDING
Can range from minor bleeding to life-threatening hemorrhage.
Consequently, factor Xa inhibitors are contraindicated in patients with active pathological bleeding.
Advise patients to report unusual bruising or bleeding to their healthcare provider.

STRESS THE IMPORTANCE *of* TAKING EXACTLY AS PRESCRIBED
Compliance is important with all medications; however, the consequence of failing to take an anticoagulant as prescribed could be fatal. An overdose could cause a life-threatening hemorrhage and missed doses could lead to a thromboembolic event.

NO ANTIDOTES/REVERSAL AGENTS
Factor Xa inhibitors are unique from all other anticoagulants as there are no known antidotes or reversal agents. Coumadin® (warfarin) has vitamin K, heparin has protamine, and Pradaxa® (dabigatran) has Praxbind® (idarucizumab), but no such antidote exists for the factor Xa inhibitors.

SPECIAL ADMINISTRATION INSTRUCTIONS *for* XARELTO® (RIVAROXABAN)
Generally, factor Xa inhibitors can be administered with or without food; however, there is one exception. Xarelto® (rivaroxaban), specifically in doses of **15 mg and 20 mg should be given with food**; however, the 10-mg dose can be given with or without food.

ORAL FACTOR Xa INHIBITORS + NSAIDs = ↑ RISK *of* GASTROINTESTINAL (GI) BLEEDING
Non-steroidal anti-inflammatory drugs (NSAIDs) have the potential to cause GI bleeding directly by irritating the GI mucosa and indirectly by reducing prostaglandin-mediated gastric mucus production. Concurrent use of a drug that interferes with coagulation (e.g. apixaban, edoxaban, rivaroxaban) increases this risk of bleeding. Unless instructed otherwise, patients on dabigatran should avoid aspirin, ibuprofen, and naproxen.

**HECKMAN'S
NURSING PHARMACOLOGY SIMPLIFIED**

HEPARIN

Mechanism: Heparin prevents the conversion of fibrinogen to fibrin, a key component of blood clots.

Common Uses: Deep vein thrombosis, pulmonary embolism, myocardial infarction

---

*Heparin blocks the conversion of fibrinogen to fibrin, but it does not dissolve fibrin. In other words, heparin prevents new blood clots and stops blood clots from growing larger but does **not** dissolve existing clots.*

ADMINISTER IV OR SQ
Heparin has a shorter duration of action and is more likely to cause pain and hematoma at the injection site when given intramuscularly. Always administer heparin by intravenous (IV) or subcutaneous (SQ) injection.

BLEEDING
Bleeding can be minor or major. Monitor for signs of bleeding such as unexplained drops in blood pressure or hematocrit. Also, advise patients to avoid non-steroidal anti-inflammatory drugs (e.g. aspirin, ibuprofen) as they increase bleeding risk.

THE ANTICOAGULANT *of* CHOICE DURING PREGNANCY
Heparin molecules are large and do not cross the placenta.

KEY MONITORING PARAMETERS

ACTIVATED PROTHROMBIN TIME (aPTT)
The anticoagulant effect of heparin must be monitored typically once every 4–6 hours, and the infusion rate must be adjusted accordingly.

PLATELET COUNT
Heparin-induced thrombocytopenia is an allergic reaction characterized by low platelets. Monitor the platelet count once every 2–3 days.

LOW MOLECULAR WEIGHT HEPARINS (LMWHs)
LMWHs, such as Lovenox® (enoxaparin), selectively inhibit the activity of factor Xa, producing a more predictable anticoagulant effect that does **not** require aPTT monitoring.

A HIGH ALERT MEDICATION

HEPARIN LOCK FLUSH: 10–100 UNITS/ML
Lower concentrations (10–100 units/mL) are used to "flush" IV catheters, preventing formation of a fibrin sheath on the tip of the IV line. These concentrations are too low for therapeutic use.

HEPARIN INJECTION: 1,000+ UNITS/ML
Higher concentrations (≥1,000 units/mL) are used therapeutically for treatment and prevention of blood clots. Never use highly concentrated heparin to flush IV lines, as doing so can be deadly.

NOTE: Erroneous administration of the incorrect concentration of heparin can have deadly consequences. Two healthcare professionals should always check the dose prior to administration.

THE ANTIDOTE *for* HEPARIN
Protamine binds to and forms a stable complex with heparin, effectively neutralizing heparin.
NOTE: 1 mg of protamine neutralizes about 100 units of heparin (or 1 mg of enoxaparin).

**HECKMAN'S
NURSING PHARMACOLOGY SIMPLIFIED**

THIENOPYRIDINES

COMMON EXAMPLES
Plavix® (clopidogrel)   Effient® (prasugrel)

Mechanism: Thienopyridines irreversibly bind to and block $P2Y_{12}$ receptors on platelets to reduce platelet aggregation and blood clot formation.

Common Uses: Prevention of myocardial infarction and stroke in patients with acute coronary syndrome (ACS), peripheral arterial disease, or recent history of heart attack or stroke

---

INHIBITION *of* PLATELET AGGREGATION

PLAVIX® (CLOPIDOGREL)	EFFIENT® (PRASUGREL)
40-60%	**70%**

Effient® (prasugrel) is more effective at preventing recurrent cardiovascular events; however, it is also more likely to cause minor and major bleeding.

THE LOADING DOSE
for PATIENTS WITH ACS
Patients with ACS typically receive a higher initial dose ("loading dose") to expedite the onset of the antiplatelet effect. The loading dose for Plavix® (clopidogrel) is a one-time dose of 300 mg, and the loading dose for Effient® (prasugrel) is a one-time dose of 60 mg. Subsequent daily doses should not exceed 75 mg for Plavix® (clopidogrel) or 10 mg for Effient® (prasugrel).

BLEEDING
THE #1 SIDE EFFECT
Bleeding is both the most common and, potentially, the most serious side effect.
This can range from something as minor as a nosebleed to major life-threatening hemorrhage.
Active bleeding (e.g. peptic ulcer, intracranial hemorrhage) is a contraindication for thienopyridines.

INCREASED RISK *of* BLEEDING WITH NSAIDs
Non-steroidal anti-inflammatory drugs (NSAIDs) irritate the stomach and increase the risk of gastrointestinal bleeding. Patients who take a thienopyridine should not take NSAIDs (e.g. aspirin, ibuprofen, naproxen) without consulting a physician; however, be aware that many patients who take a thienopyridine should also be taking a once-daily dose of aspirin for the added antiplatelet effect, despite the increased risk of bleeding.

THROMBOTIC THROMBOCYTOPENIC PURPURA (TTP)
TTP is a potentially fatal adverse reaction characterized by purple spots (purpura) on the skin or in the mouth.
Other findings include low platelets, fragmented red blood cells, kidney dysfunction, and fever.

HECKMAN'S
NURSING PHARMACOLOGY SIMPLIFIED

BILE ACID RESINS

COMMON EXAMPLES
Questran® (cholestyramine)   Colestid® (colestipol)

Mechanism: Bile acid resins bind and remove bile acids from the gastrointestinal (GI) tract by way of the stool, forcing the liver to produce new bile acids.

Common Uses: High cholesterol

THE BILE ACID-CHOLESTEROL RELATIONSHIP
Bile acids are hepatically synthesized from cholesterol and secreted into the GI tract to aid in the digestion of fats. Normally, bile acids are reabsorbed from the GI tract and reused; however, when we remove the bile acids, the liver compensates by producing more, ultimately lowering cholesterol.

ADMINISTER BEFORE A MEAL
Bile acid secretion spikes when food enters the GI tract, so administer before a meal for best results.

INSTRUCT PATIENTS TO DRINK QUESTRAN® QUICKLY
Questran® (cholestyramine), a powder for oral suspension, must be mixed in 2–6 ounces of non-carbonated liquid prior to administration. Questran® (cholestyramine) can damage the enamel of the teeth, causing discoloration and decay. To avoid this, instruct patients to drink the Questran® suspension **quickly**.

SIDE EFFECTS *of* BILE ACID RESINS
Bile acid resins are large polymers that are not significantly absorbed from the GI tract. Since they remain within the GI tract, this is where most of the side effects occur.

✓Constipation   ✓Abdominal discomfort   ✓Bloating   ✓Flatulence   ✓Nausea/vomiting

NOTE: Constipation is so common that bile acid resins are sometimes used off-label to treat diarrhea.

↑ FLUIDS + ↑ FIBER ± STOOL SOFTENER
Encourage the patient to increase fluid and fiber intake (e.g. water and Metamucil®) to address bile acid resin-induced constipation. A stool softener (e.g. Colace®) can also be added, if necessary.

VITAMIN DEFICIENCIES
Bile acids aid in the digestion of fats and fat-soluble vitamins. Unsurprisingly, fat-soluble vitamin deficiencies (A, D, E, and K) can occur with the long-term use of bile acid resins.

DRUG INTERACTIONS
Because they are binding agents, bile acid resins interact with just about everything. Administer other medications at least one hour before or 4–6 hours after bile acid resins to avoid interactions.

HECKMAN'S
NURSING PHARMACOLOGY SIMPLIFIED

HMG-CoA REDUCTASE INHIBITORS

COMMON EXAMPLES
Lipitor® (atorvastatin)   Crestor® (rosuvastatin)
Zocor® (simvastatin)   Pravachol® (pravastatin)   Mevacor® (lovastatin)

Drug Name Stem: –statin

Mechanism: HMG-CoA reductase inhibitors block the key enzyme involved in the biological production of cholesterol.

Common Uses: High cholesterol

SPECIAL ADMINISTRATION INSTRUCTIONS

ADMINISTER IN THE EVENING
Generally, statins work best when given in the evening, probably because hepatic production of cholesterol peaks during the night; however, time of administration is not clinically significant for atorvastatin, rosuvastatin, or pravastatin. These statins can be given at any time.

AVOID GRAPEFRUIT JUICE
Certain compounds in grapefruit juice is known to inhibit the key enzyme (CYP3A4) involved in the elimination of atorvastatin, lovastatin, and simvastatin. Consuming grapefruit juice while taking one of these three statins increases the risk of side effects such as myopathy and rhabdomyolysis.

ADMINISTER WITH *or* WITHOUT FOOD
Generally, food does not enhance or interfere with the absorption of statins. The exception is Mevacor® (lovastatin), which should be given once daily with the evening meal.

SERIOUS ADVERSE EFFECTS

SKELETAL MUSCLE TOXICITY
Statins can cause myopathy. In severe cases, life-threating rhabdomyolysis may occur.
↓
Advise patients to report unexplained muscle pain or weakness to their physician.

LIVER TOXICITY
Patients should get baseline liver function tests with follow-up testing as necessary.
↓
Monitor for fatigue, dark urine, abdominal pain, nausea, appetite loss, and jaundice.

PREGNANCY CATEGORY X
Babies need cholesterol for normal development, so
statins should never be used in women who are pregnant or nursing.

FIBRATES

COMMON EXAMPLES
Lopid® (gemfibrozil)   Tricor® (fenofibrate)

Drug Name Stem: –fibr–

Mechanism: Fibrates promote lipolysis and the elimination of triglycerides from the bloodstream.

Common Uses: Hyperlipidemia with high triglycerides

LOPID® (GEMFIBROZIL)
Administer 30 minutes before a meal.

TRICOR® (FENOFIBRATE)
Administer with or without food.

TRIGLYCERIDE REDUCTION
Fibrates are used specifically to treat certain types of hyperlipidemia involving high triglyceride levels.

GASTROINTESTINAL SIDE EFFECTS
The most common side effects of Lopid® (gemfibrozil) can be categorized broadly as gastrointestinal side effects and include dyspepsia, abdominal pain, diarrhea, nausea, and vomiting. Abdominal pain and nausea are also common side effects of Tricor® (fenofibrate).

SERIOUS ADVERSE EFFECTS

SKELETAL MUSCLE TOXICITY
Like the HMG-CoA reductase inhibitors ("statins"), fibrates are also associated with myopathy and rhabdomyolysis (i.e. muscle toxicity). The risk is higher for elderly patients and patients on a statin. Advise patients to report unexplained muscle pain or weakness to their physician.

LIVER TOXICITY
Liver function abnormalities are a common side effect of fibrates. Patients should receive baseline liver function tests prior to starting a fibrate, and periodic liver function tests as treatment continues. Monitor for fatigue, dark urine, abdominal pain, nausea, appetite loss, and jaundice.

COMMON DRUG INTERACTIONS

FIBRATE + STATIN
As mentioned previously, the risk of myopathy and rhabdomyolysis is higher in patients who are also taking a statin drug (e.g. atorvastatin, lovastatin, rosuvastatin, simvastatin).

FIBRATE + WARFARIN
Fibrates interfere with the metabolism of warfarin by the liver. Consequently, INR levels can be expected to increase when a fibrate drug is initiated in a patient on warfarin.

HECKMAN'S
NURSING PHARMACOLOGY SIMPLIFIED

NON-STEROIDAL ANTI-INFLAMMATORY DRUGS

COMMON EXAMPLES
Motrin®, Advil® (ibuprofen)   Naprosyn®, Aleve® (naproxen)   Indocin (indomethacin)
Mobic® (meloxicam)   Voltaren® (diclofenac)   Toradol® (ketorolac)   aspirin

Mechanism: Non-steroidal anti-inflammatory drugs (NSAIDs) reduce prostaglandin synthesis by inhibiting cyclooxygenase enzymes (COX-1 & 2), which ultimately produces analgesic and antipyretic effects.
Common Uses: Mild–moderate pain, fever, inflammation

NSAIDs *for* DYSMENORRHEA
Endogenously-produced prostaglandins increase intrauterine pressure and stimulate contractions during menstruation. In some cases, this can cause painful cramps. NSAIDs reduce prostaglandin synthesis, ultimately reducing intrauterine pressure and decreasing the frequency of uterine contractions.

POTENTIALLY DEADLY SIDE EFFECTS *of* NSAIDs

GASTROINTESTINAL IRRITATION
NSAIDs increase the risk of gastrointestinal bleeding, ulceration, and perforation. Monitor for signs and symptoms of gastrointestinal bleeding and administer NSAIDs with food to reduce gastrointestinal irritation.

CARDIOVASCULAR EVENTS
NSAIDs increase the risk of cardiovascular events, such as heart attack and stroke. They can also elevate blood pressure and blunt the effects of blood pressure-lowering medications. Monitor blood pressure periodically.

AVOID NSAIDs DURING THE THIRD TRIMESTER *of* PREGNANCY
Use of NSAIDs by women ≥ 30 weeks pregnant can cause premature closure of the fetal ductus arteriosus, a potentially deadly cardiovascular defect.

THREE UNIQUE NSAIDs

CELEBREX® (CELECOXIB)
Relatively gentle on the stomach. Other NSAIDs indiscriminately inhibit COX-1 and COX-2. Celebrex® is unique in that it selectively inhibits COX-2. This is impactful because it preserves the activity of COX-1, which plays a role in protecting the lining of the stomach from the corrosive effects of gastric acid.

TORADOL® (KETOROLAC)
The most powerful NSAID. While other NSAIDs can be used for mild–moderate pain, Toradol® is approved for moderately severe acute pain; however, this power comes with drawbacks. Toradol® should only be used short-term (**no more than five days**) due to higher risk of potentially deadly gastrointestinal bleeding and renal toxicity.

ASPIRIN
Aspirin irreversibly inhibits cyclooxygenase, producing a stronger antiplatelet effect compared to other NSAIDs. Consequently, aspirin can be used daily to prevent cardiovascular events such as heart attack and stroke. The use of aspirin by children or teenagers who are recovering from a viral infection, such as the chickenpox, influenza, or the common cold, is associated with Reye's syndrome. Although Reye's syndrome is rare, a high percentage of cases are fatal. To be prudent, avoid the use of aspirin in all patients ≤ 19 years-old.

HECKMAN'S
NURSING PHARMACOLOGY SIMPLIFIED

COAL TAR-DERIVED ANALGESICS

THE MOST COMMON EXAMPLE
Tylenol® (acetaminophen)

Mechanism: Acetaminophen appears to inhibit cyclooxygenase only in the central nervous system.

Common Uses: Pain, fever

THE ABBREVIATION for ACETAMINOPHEN
APAP, the abbreviation for acetaminophen is derived from the chemical name: n-**a**cetyl **p**-**a**mino **p**henol

A COMPARISON of ACETAMINOPHEN VERSUS NSAIDs

	Acetaminophen	NSAIDs
Analgesic-Antipyretic Effect	Moderate	Moderate
Anti-inflammatory Effect	Weak	Strong
Antiplatelet Effect	No	Yes
Gastric Irritation	No	Yes

As shown above, acetaminophen does not increase the risk of bleeding or gastric ulceration, but at the expense of meaningful anti-inflammatory activity.

THE DRUG OF CHOICE for PAIN DURING PREGNANCY
Acetaminophen is considered safe during pregnancy when used as directed. Unlike NSAIDs, acetaminophen does not inhibit prostaglandin synthesis and consequently will not cause premature closure of the ductus arteriosus when used in the third trimester of pregnancy.

4,000 MG MAXIMUM DAILY DOSE
An overdose of acetaminophen can cause liver failure and death, particularly with doses in excess of 4,000 mg per day (or 3,000 mg per day for elderly patients).

INSTRUCT PATIENTS TO AVOID ALCOHOL
NOTE: Drinking alcohol while taking acetaminophen can cause severe, potentially fatal liver damage.

COMBINATION PRODUCTS
Acetaminophen is found in numerous combination products for pain and the common cold, heightening the risk of unintentional overdose. To ensure patients do not exceed the maximum daily dose, keep track of acetaminophen taken from all sources. See below for select examples of combination products.

Over-The-Counter Products	Prescription Only Products
Tylenol®, Excedrin®, DayQuil™, Theraflu®	Percocet®, Vicodin®, Ultracet®, Tylenol® #3

THE ANTIDOTE for ACETAMINOPHEN
Acetadote® (acetylcysteine)

HECKMAN'S
NURSING PHARMACOLOGY SIMPLIFIED

OPIOID ANALGESICS

COMMON EXAMPLES
morphine   codeine   hydrocodone   oxycodone
hydromorphone   oxymorphone   fentanyl   methadone

Mechanism: Opioids activate μ (mu)-opioid receptors in the nervous system, producing analgesia.
Common Uses: Moderate–severe pain

THE OPIUM POPPY PLANT
Morphine and codeine are compounds derived directly from the opium poppy. Hydro**morph**one and oxy**morph**one are semi-synthetic derivatives of morphine. Hydro**cod**one and oxy**cod**one are semi-synthetic derivatives of codeine. Opioids like fentanyl and methadone are fully synthetic (man-made).

CONTROLLED SUBSTANCES
All opioid analgesics are categorized as controlled substances due to their potential for abuse and addiction.

UNDESIRED ACTIVITY and SIDE EFFECTS

ACTIVITY	EFFECT
Stimulation of the chemoreceptor trigger zone	Nausea/vomiting
Dilation of peripheral blood vessels	Hypotension, flushing, itching
Depression of central nervous system activity	Sedation, respiratory depression
Depression of intestinal peristaltic activity	Constipation

NOTE: Patients frequently self-report nausea/vomiting and itching as "allergic reactions." When the patient says they are allergic to any medication, document the details of the reaction so we can differentiate between side effects and allergies.

SEDATION and LIFE-THREATENING RESPIRATORY DEPRESSION
Higher doses of an opioid produce a greater analgesic effect but with greater potential for sedation and respiratory depression. Monitor respiratory rate, especially when starting or increasing the dose. Also advise patients to avoid taking other depressants (including alcohol) and to avoid driving until the effects are known.

OPIOID TOLERANCE
Due to the development of tolerance, a high-dose opioid taken by an opioid-tolerant patient (i.e. one who regularly takes opioids) may cause little sedation and respiratory depression; whereas the same dose taken by a person who is opioid naïve (i.e. one who does not regularly take opioids) may be deadly. For this reason, high-dose or highly potent opioids should only be given to patients who have developed a certain level of tolerance. Examples include any dose of Duragesic® (fentanyl patch), Oxycontin® (oxycodone ER) at doses greater than 40 mg twice daily, and Nucynta® ER (tapentadol ER) at doses greater than 50 mg twice daily.

OPIOID-INDUCED CONSTIPATION
As the dose of the opioid increases, constipation worsens. Chronic opioid users usually need daily laxatives.

THE ANTIDOTE for OPIOIDS
Narcan® (naloxone), an opioid receptor antagonist.

THE END

★★★★ THANK YOU! ★★★★

Thank you for using my study guide! It actually took me years to write this book, not because it's particularly long. On the contrary, because I wanted to create something that is both ultra-brief and ultra-helpful. I hope that's the way it's perceived, but either way, I'd love to hear your thoughts! Whether positive or negative, please visit Amazon to leave a brief, honest review. I read them all, and I look forward to reading yours!

Kind regards,
David Heckman, PharmD

PLEASE LEAVE A REVIEW AT AMAZON.COM

CONTROLLED SUBSTANCE SCHEDULES

	Rx	OTC	ABUSE & DEPENDENCE	EXAMPLE
SCHEDULE I (C-I)			HIGH	HEROIN
SCHEDULE II (C-II)	✓		HIGH	ROXICODONE® OXYCODONE
SCHEDULE III (C-III)	✓		MODERATE	ANDROGEL® TESTOSTERONE
SCHEDULE IV (C-IV)	✓		MILD	VALIUM® DIAZEPAM
SCHEDULE V (C-V)	✓	✓*	LOW	CHERATUSSIN® AC GUAIFENESIN WITH CODEINE

*Limited quantities of certain C-V controlled substances may be dispensed without a prescription if state law permits.

HECKMAN'S
NURSING PHARMACOLOGY SIMPLIFIED

GENERIC DRUG NAME INDEX

acetaminophen, 108
acetylcysteine, 108
acyclovir, 22
adalimumab, 36
albuterol, 39
alendronate, 34
allopurinol, 35
alprazolam, 51
aluminum hydroxide, 67
amikacin, 16
aminophylline, 43
amiodarone, 95
amitriptyline, 58
amlodipine, 92
amoxicillin, 10
amphetamine, 54
ampicillin, 10
anastrozole, 82
apixaban, 101
aripiprazole, 62
aspirin, 107
atenolol, 89
atorvastatin, 105
atropine, 28, 44, 45, 66
azithromycin, 14

baclofen, 53
benazepril, 88
benztropine, 44
bisacodyl, 65
bisoprolol, 89
budesonide, 41
bumetanide, 85
bupropion, 57

calcium carbonate, 67
canagliflozin, 74
carbamazepine, 48
carbidopa/levodopa, 46
carboplatin, 30
carisoprodol, 53
carvedilol, 89
cefaclor, 11
cefazolin, 11
cefdinir, 11
cefepime, 11
ceftaroline, 11
ceftriaxone, 11
cefuroxime, 11
cephalexin, 11
cetirizine, 38

chlorpromazine, 61
cholestyramine, 104
cimetidine, 69
ciprofloxacin, 18
cisplatin, 30
citalopram, 55
clarithromycin, 14
clindamycin, 13
clonazepam, 51
clonidine, 91
clopidogrel, 103
clozapine, 62
codeine, 109
colchicine, 35
colestipol, 104
cyclobenzaprine, 53
cyclophosphamide, 31
cyclosporine, 37

dabigatran, 100
dapagliflozin, 74
darunavir, 24
daunorubicin, 29
deferoxamine, 33
desvenlafaxine, 56
dexamethasone, 83
dexlansoprazole, 68
dexmethylphenidate, 54
dextroamphetamine, 54
diazepam, 51
diclofenac, 107
dicloxacillin, 10
dicyclomine, 44
digoxin, 96
digoxin immune fab, 96
diltiazem, 92
dimenhydrinate, 38
diphenhydramine, 38
diphenoxylate/atropine, 66
dobutamine, 98
docetaxel, 25
docusate, 65
dolutegravir, 24
donepezil, 45
dopamine, 98
doxazosin, 90
doxepin, 58
doxorubicin, 29
doxycycline, 15
doxylamine, 38
dulaglutide, 75

duloxetine, 56
dutasteride, 79

edoxaban, 101
efavirenz, 24
empagliflozin, 74
enalapril, 88
enfuvirtide, 24
enoxaparin, 102
epinephrine, 98
epoetin alfa, 32
erythromycin, 14
escitalopram, 55
esomeprazole, 68
eszopiclone, 52
etanercept, 36
ethacrynic acid, 85
ethinyl estradiol, 80
etonogestrel, 80
exemestane, 82
exenatide, 75

famotidine, 69
febuxostat, 35
fenofibrate, 106
fentanyl, 109
ferrous fumarate, 33
ferrous gluconate, 33
ferrous sulfate, 33
fexofenadine, 38
finasteride, 79
fluconazole, 21
fludrocortisone, 84
flumazenil, 51
fluoxetine, 55
fluticasone, 41
formoterol, 39
furosemide, 85

gabapentin, 49
gemfibrozil, 106
gentamicin, 16
glimepiride, 74
glipizide, 74
glucagon, 72
glyburide, 74
granisetron, 64

haloperidol, 61
heparin, 102
hydrochlorothiazide, 86

hydrocodone, 109
hydrocortisone, 83
hydromorphone, 109
hyoscyamine, 44

ibandronate, 34
ibuprofen, 107
idarubicin, 29
idarucizumab, 100
imipramine, 58
indomethacin, 107
infliximab, 36
insulin, 72
ipratropium, 40
irbesartan, 88
irinotecan, 28
iron, 33
isocarboxazid, 59
isosorbide, 93

ketoconazole, 21
ketorolac, 107

labetalol, 89
lactulose, 65
lansoprazole, 68
letrozole, 82
leucovorin, 27
levalbuterol, 39
levodopa/carbidopa, 46
levofloxacin, 18
levomilnacipran, 56
levonorgestrel, 81
levothyroxine, 76
lidocaine, 95
linagliptin, 74
linezolid, 20
liraglutide, 75
lisdexamfetamine, 54
lisinopril, 88
loperamide, 66
loratadine, 38
lorazepam, 51
losartan, 88
lovastatin, 105

magnesium carbonate, 67
magnesium hydroxide, 65
magnesium hydroxide, 67
maraviroc, 24
medroxyprogesterone, 81
meloxicam, 107
metformin, 73
methadone, 109
methicillin, 10

methimazole, 77
methotrexate, 27
methylcellulose, 65
methyldopa, 91
methylphenidate, 54
methylprednisolone, 83
metoclopramide, 63
metoprolol, 89
metronidazole, 9
milnacipran, 56
misoprostol, 71
mometasone, 41
montelukast, 42
morphine, 109
moxifloxacin, 18

nafcillin, 10
naloxone, 109
naproxen, 107
nebivolol, 89
nevirapine, 24
nicardipine, 92
nifedipine, 92
nitrofurantoin, 12
nitroglycerin, 93
norelgestromin, 80
norepinephrine, 98
norethindrone, 81
norgestimate, 80
nortriptyline, 58

olanzapine, 62
olmesartan, 88
omeprazole, 68
ondansetron, 64
oseltamivir, 23
oxacillin, 10
oxaliplatin, 30
oxybutynin, 44
oxycodone, 109
oxymorphone, 109

paclitaxel, 25
palonosetron, 64
pantoprazole, 68
paroxetine, 55
penicillin, 10
phenelzine, 59
phenobarbital, 50
phenylephrine, 98
phenytoin, 48
physostigmine, 44
phytonadione, 99
pioglitazone, 74
piperacillin, 10

polycarbophil, 65
polyethylene glycol, 65
polystyrene sulfonate, 97
potassium chloride, 97
pramipexole, 47
prasugrel, 103
pravastatin, 105
prazosin, 90
prednisolone, 83
prednisone, 83
pregabalin, 49
propranolol, 89
propylthiouracil, 77
protamine, 102
psyllium fiber, 65

quetiapine, 62

raltegravir, 24
ramipril, 88
ranitidine, 69
risedronate, 34
risperidone, 62
ritonavir, 24
rivaroxaban, 101
rivastigmine, 45
rizatriptan, 60
ropinirole, 47
rosiglitazone, 74
rosuvastatin, 105

salmeterol, 39
sennosides, 65
sertraline, 55
sildenafil, 94
silodosin, 90
simethicone, 67
simvastatin, 105
sitagliptin, 74
solifenacin, 44
sotalol, 89, 95
spironolactone, 87
sucralfate, 70
sulfamethoxazole, 19
sumatriptan, 60

tacrolimus, 37
tadalafil, 94
tamsulosin, 90
temazepam, 51
tenofovir, 24
terazosin, 90
testosterone, 78
tetracycline, 15
theophylline, 43

ticarcillin, 10
tiotropium, 40
tizanidine, 91
tobramycin, 16
tolterodine, 44
topotecan, 28
torsemide, 85
tranylcypromine, 59
trazodone, 55
triazolam, 51
trihexyphenidyl, 44

trimethoprim, 19

valacyclovir, 22
valproic acid, 48
valsartan, 88
vancomycin, 17
vardenafil, 94
venlafaxine, 56
verapamil, 92
vinblastine, 26
vincristine, 26

warfarin, 99

zafirlukast, 42
zaleplon, 52
zidovudine, 24
ziprasidone, 62
zolmitriptan, 60
zolpidem, 52

Made in the USA
Las Vegas, NV
22 October 2024

10283707R00066